Sex- and Gender-Based Analysis in Public Health

Jacqueline Gahagan • Mary K. Bryson
Editors

Sex- and Gender-Based Analysis in Public Health

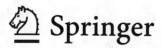 Springer

Editors
Jacqueline Gahagan
Faculty of Health
Dalhousie University
Halifax, NS
Canada

Mary K. Bryson
Department of Language and Literacy
Education, Faculty of Education
University of British Columbia
Vancouver, BC
Canada

ISBN 978-3-030-71931-9   ISBN 978-3-030-71929-6   (eBook)
https://doi.org/10.1007/978-3-030-71929-6

This Springer imprint is published by the registered company Springer Nature Switzerland AG
The registered company address is: Gewerbestrasse 11, 6330 Cham, Switzerland

Foreword

At the World Health Organization (WHO), we operate with the core assumption that sex- and gender-based analysis (SGBA) can help us: (a) better understand conditions faced by women, men, transgender and gender-diverse people, and (b) tailor appropriately the effects that policies may have on marginalized populations. Specifically, SGBA can tell us who has access and who benefits from public health policies and who is likely to be missed. It sheds light on social and structural determinants of health that help us focus our efforts within or outside complex health systems.

The WHO is committed to sex- and gender-based analysis for these reasons. Perhaps most importantly, sex- and gender-based analysis should not take place in isolation from other modes of intersectional equity-focused modes of analysis. For example, disaggregation of health data by a range of linked and relevant determinants of health equity, such as wealth, geographic location, age, and ethnicity, among others, provides a more robust portrayal of people's lives and situations. Traditionally, public health has leaned towards looking at aggregate levels of impact, as a macro lens provides a powerful population-level analysis. However, without understanding which groups are being missed through disaggregation, we are not able to address the sex- and gender-based barriers that must be prioritized to see population-specific shifts in health disparities.

Public health trainees and the larger public health community need conceptual clarity regarding what are biological, what are social, and what are structural contributors to poor health outcomes. In many instances we may see a combination of the above. For example, men may be more biologically susceptible to tuberculosis, but gender-normative behaviors understood as harmful masculinities such as avoiding healthcare services and smoking must be considered as well. Structural forces and inequalities continue to contribute to a variety of health and social disparities, including poverty, working conditions, and globalization through migration and discrimination.

Gender is a contested and relational concept and one that should not be analyzed in isolation. While many cisgender or transgender women around the world are in relationships with men who are brothers, sons, husbands, and employers, they experience different treatment under social- and health-related structures. We also know that men tend to die earlier and women live longer on average but with more chronic diseases. When men, for example, in the household die earlier, women are often burdened with unpaid care work when they are unwell and larger out-of-pocket expenses leading to economic and social disenfranchisement. As such, we must disaggregate by sex and conduct gender analysis that includes women and men, as well as transgender and gender-diverse groups no matter which group carries a heavier burden while also examining these relational aspects.

This book on sex- and gender-based analysis in public health provides an opportunity for trainees entering the field of public health to build skills and perspectives on how to approach complex public health problems with a lens towards fairness and justice. By avoiding the limitation of data which are not, for example, disaggregated by sex or by gender, we will be better able to offer a more nuanced understanding of how to ensure our public health programs, interventions, and policies are able to demonstrate impact and effectiveness. It is vitally important, therefore, that our public health approach does not sacrifice equity for efficiency. This approach heralds the beginning of a new sex- and gender-based analytic era in public health, one that is committed to reducing disparities and related poor health outcomes.

Veronica Magar
Director, Gender, Equity and Human Rights
World Health Organization (WHO)
Geneva, Switzerland

Contents

Contributors

Catrine Andersson, PhD Centre for Sexology and Sexuality Studies, Department of Social Work, Faculty of Health and Society, Malmö University, Malmö, Sweden

Mary K. Bryson, PhD Department of Language and Literacy Education, Faculty of Education, University of British Columbia, Vancouver, BC, Canada

Allison Carter, PhD Kirby Institute, University of New South Wales, Sydney, NSW, Australia

Faculty of Health Sciences, Simon Fraser University, Burnaby, BC, Canada

Jeremiah Chikovore, PhD Human and Social Capabilities Research Division, Human Sciences Research Council, Durban, South Africa

Natisha Dukhi, PhD Human and Social Capabilities, Human Sciences Research Council, Pretoria, South Africa

Shari L. Dworkin, PhD, MS School of Nursing and Health Studies, University of Washington Bothell, Bothell, WA, USA

Karyn Fulcher, PhD School of Public Health and Social Policy, University of Victoria, Victoria, BC, Canada

Jacqueline Gahagan, PhD Faculty of Health, Dalhousie University, Halifax, NS, Canada

Lorraine Greaves, PhD Centre of Excellence for Women's Health, Vancouver, BC, Canada

Olena Hankivsky, PhD Centre for Health Equity, Melbourne School of Population and Global Health, University of Melbourne, Carlton, VIC, Australia

Shirin Heidari, PhD GENDRO, Geneva, Switzerland

Global Health Centre, Graduate Institute of International and Development Studies, Geneva, Switzerland

Natalie Hemsing, MA Centre of Excellence for Women's Health, Vancouver, BC, Canada

Gemma Hunting, MA International Health Equity Consultant, Coburg, Bavaria, Germany

Nathan Lachowsky, PhD School of Public Health and Social Policy, University of Victoria, Victoria, BC, Canada

Community-Based Research Centre, Vancouver, BC, Canada

Malin Lindroth, PhD Centre for Sexology and Sexuality Studies, Department of Social Work, Faculty of Health and Society, Malmö University, Malmö, Sweden

Sizulu Moyo, MBChB, MPH, PhD Human Sciences Research Council, Human and Social Capabilities Programme, Cape Town, South Africa

School of Public Health, University of Cape Town, Cape Town, South Africa

Olanrewaju Oladimeji, PhD Department of Global Health and Population, Harvard T.H. Chan School of Public Health, Boston, MA, USA

Nancy Poole, PhD Centre of Excellence for Women's Health, Vancouver, BC, Canada

CanFASD Research Network, Vancouver, BC, Canada

Priscilla Reddy, PhD Human and Social Capabilities, Human Sciences Research Council, Pretoria, South Africa

Cara Tannenbaum, MD, MSc Faculty of Medicine, Université de Montréal, Montreal, QC, Canada

Krystle van Hoof, MA Healthy Brains, Healthy Lives, McGill University, Montreal, QC, Canada

Fiona Warde, MD Department of Family Medicine, Queen's University, Kingston, ON, Canada

Nompumelelo Zungu, PhD Human Sciences Research Council, Pretoria, South Africa

Human and Social Capabilities, Human Sciences Research Council, Pretoria, South Africa

Department of Psychology, University of Pretoria, Pretoria, South Africa

About the Editors

Jacqueline (Jacquie) Gahagan, PhD, is a medical sociologist and a Full Professor of Health Promotion in the Faculty of Health at Dalhousie University, Halifax, Nova Scotia, Canada. Jacquie teaches program planning, measurement, and evaluation and serves as the Co-Director of the Atlantic Interdisciplinary Research Network for Social and Behavioural Aspects of HIV and HCV (airn.ca), which is an Atlantic regional network of over 250 researchers, policy-makers, and community-based service providers. Jacquie holds Research Associate positions with the Jean Monnet European Union Centre of Excellence, the Health Law Institute, and the Beatrice Hunter Cancer Research Institute, is a Founding Fellow of the MacEachen Institute for Public Policy and Governance, and is an Affiliate Scientist with the Nova Scotia Health Authority.

Jacquie's program of mixed-methods health promotion research focuses on evaluating policy and programming interventions using sex- and gender-based analyses (SGBA+) to address health inequities among marginalized populations including those living with or affected by HIV, HCV, or other STBBIs, the scaling-up of access to innovative HIV testing technologies, older LGBTQ2I populations and housing, primary healthcare utilization among LGBTQ2I communities, and end-of-life decision-making. Prior to joining Dalhousie University, Jacquie worked as an evaluation specialist in public health at the municipal, provincial, and national levels in relation to harm reduction, HIV/HCV prevention, and tobacco use cessation.

Mary K. Bryson, PhD, is Senior Associate Dean, Administration, Faculty Affairs & Innovation and Professor, Department of Language and Literacy Education, Faculty of Education, University of British Columbia in Vancouver, BC, Canada. Dr. Bryson's program of research is designed so as to contribute foundational scholarship concerning access to knowledge, gender, and sexual marginality and resilience, and in so doing, to make significant contributions to a growing archive that documents the social, cultural, and educational significance of networked media technologies and publics. A hallmark of the trajectory of their funded research projects is to contribute evidence concerning sexuality and gender, and the role of networked social media and information literacies that shape access to knowledge and its mobilization. Their leadership in theory-building in the areas of cognition, agency, and digital culture have proven invaluable in framing humanistic models of digital and epistemic competencies particularly relevant to complex minority cultures in the twenty-first century. Vital to their contributions are Dr. Bryson's innovative and career-long contributions in the area of intersectionality, minority stress, and non-deterministic ways of thinking about the significance of digital media and networks to members of minority groups. The Cancer's Margins project that Dr. Bryson directs (www.lgbtcancer.ca) is Canada's first CIHR-funded national investigation of sexual and gender marginality and access to/mobilization of cancer knowledge.

About the Contributors

Catrine Andersson, PhD, is associate professor in social work and teaches the master's program in sexology at Malmö University in Sweden. Andersson's research is focused on norms of coupledom, non-monogamous practices, love, family, and sexuality. Ongoing projects involve, for example, research on infidelity, where life stories on experiences of infidelity between 1940 and 2020 are collected digitally. Recent publications include "Non-monogamous parenthood: recognition and legitimacy beyond norms of coupledom" published in *lambda Nordica* (2019) and "Living outside of protocol – Polyamorous orientations, bodies and queer temporalities" published in *Sexuality & Culture* (2019).

Allison Carter, PhD, is a lecturer with the Kirby Institute at the University of New South Wales in Australia and an Adjunct Professor in the Faculty of Health Sciences at Simon Fraser University in Canada. Her research program focuses on the intersections of gender, society, and sexual and reproductive health and rights, particularly for communities that are less well-represented in sexuality research and social policy.

Jeremiah Chikovore, PhD, is a Senior Research Specialist in the Human and Social Capabilities research division at the Human Sciences Research Council (HSRC) in Durban, South Africa. Dr. Chikovore holds a BSc (Hons.) from the University of Zimbabwe, and a Master's in Public Health and PhD in Public Health, both from Umea University in Sweden. Dr. Chikovore has been working in the area of public health using a social sciences lens for the past two decades, primarily in the fields of TB, HIV and AIDS, and sexual and reproductive health, and largely applying gendered and masculinity-based analyses. Dr. Chikovore has led, directed, and served as co-investigator on various studies, working in collaboration with local, regional, and international partners. A former Wellcome Trust Training Fellow, Dr. Chikovore regularly provides expert advice to various international bodies.

Natisha Dukhi, PhD, is a Research Specialist at the Human Sciences Research Council in South Africa. She has over a decade of experience as a Medical Scientist, specializing in Human Anatomy, Physiology, Pathophysiology, and Nutrition. In 2015, she completed her PhD in Public Health at the University of KwaZulu-Natal in South Africa. She is an eclectic behavioral scientist, with various interdisciplinary research focuses. These include Maternal, Adolescent and Child Health, with specific niche areas such as non-communicable diseases, mHealth, artificial intelligence in Health, nutrition and gender-based violence. She is on the Executive Board of Directors for the Public Health Association of South Africa (PHASA), Affiliate Member of the African Academy of Sciences (AAS), and President of the African ChangeMakers South African chapter, among others. In 2018, she was a BRICS Young Scientist awardee and a recipient of the Gro Brundtland Award for outstanding work in the field of public health and sustainable development.

Shari L. Dworkin, PhD, MS, is Dean and Professor in the School of Nursing and Health Studies at the University of Washington Bothell in the USA. Her research is focused on gender relations and HIV prevention, treatment, and care. Her research is also focused on masculinities-based gender-transformative HIV and family planning interventions. She is the author or co-author of over 90 peer-reviewed journal articles and 3 books, including *Men at Risk: Masculinities, Heterosexuality and HIV Prevention* (NYU Press). She is the Co-Editor of *Women's Empowerment and Global Health: A 21st Century Agenda* (UC Press). Dr. Dworkin is Associate Editor at the *Archives of Sexual Behavior* and is the current President of the International Academy of Sex Research.

Karyn Fulcher, PhD, is a Postdoctoral Fellow in the School of Public Health and Social Policy at the University of Victoria in Australia. She has conducted interdisciplinary and community-based research in Australia and Canada, drawing on her background in biology, anthropology, and sexuality and relationships education. Karyn uses qualitative and mixed-methods approaches to better understand the sexual healthcare and education needs of young people and sexual and gender minorities, in order to inform the provision of inclusive and appropriate sexual health education and health services.

Lorraine Greaves, PhD, is a medical sociologist and Senior Investigator at the Centre of Excellence for Women's Health in Vancouver, British Columbia, Canada, and founder and past president of the International Network of Women Against Tobacco. She researches sex and gender and their impact on women's health, particularly tobacco use, substance use, opioids, violence, and trauma, and has designed numerous practical products to improve health information, healthcare provision, and sex-, gender-, and equity-based analysis. She is the author of 12 books and numerous articles and reports, and a frequent speaker. A recipient of numerous awards, including a YWCA Woman of Distinction Award and an honorary doctorate from the University of Ottawa, she has been named to the Canadian Women in Global Health List, is part of the Scientific Advisory Board on Vaping Products, and chairs the Scientific Advisory Committee on Health Products for Women for Health Canada.

Olena Hankivsky, PhD, is Research Chair and Gender and Equity Director at the Centre for Health Equity, Melbourne School of Population and Global Health, University of Melbourne, Australia, is trained as a political scientist. She has been a Canadian Institutes of Health Research Chair in Gender and Health Research and a Michael Smith Foundation for Health Research Senior Scholar in Population Health (2009–2014), as well as a Visiting Professor at Columbia University Mailman School of Public Health in New York (2008–2009) and the London School of Hygiene and Tropical Medicine (2014–2015). She has led the development of gender-based analysis plus (GBA+) policy for Status of Women Canada (2012), and an intersectionality-based analysis framework for health inequities (2012). Dr. Hankivsky edited the collection *Health Inequities in Canada: Intersectional Frameworks and Practices* (UBC Press, 2011), and co-edited *Women's Health in Canada* (2007, 2nd edition forthcoming). She has conducted mixed-method research in countries including Ukraine, the United Kingdom, Sweden, Australia, Colombia, India, and Canada.

Shirin Heidari, PhD, is the founding president of GENDRO, an association with the mission to advance gender-sensitive research. She is also Senior Researcher at Global Health Centre, and research affiliate of Gender Centre, at the Graduate Institute of International and Development Studies in Geneva, Switzerland.

Dr. Heidari received her doctorate at Karolinska Institute in Sweden in 2001, where she continued as HIV researcher until her move to Geneva in 2007. She has held senior leadership positions in International AIDS Society and Reproductive Health Matters and been a board member of Amnesty International, Sweden. She is the founding chair of the Gender Policy Committee of the European Association of Science Editors (EASE), where she led the development of the Sex and Gender Equity in Research (SAGER) guidelines. She has given a TEDx talk encouraging gender-sensitive research and scholarly communication.

Natalie Hemsing, MA, is a Research Associate at the Centre of Excellence for Women's Health in Vancouver, British Columbia, Canada. She has an extensive background in: sex- and gender-based analysis; smoking prevention, cessation, and tobacco policy among diverse populations; gender and substance use; and systematic reviews and knowledge syntheses.

Gemma Hunting, MA, is an international health equity consultant working to promote equity within health research, policy, and practice. Areas of expertise include: Indigenous health, gender mainstreaming, and health equity frameworks. She has worked for national and international government bodies, organizations, and universities, including: the Gender, Equity and Human Rights Team and Mental Health Team (WHO), the International Institute for Global Health (UN University),

UN Women, the National Collaborating Centre for Determinants of Health in Canada, the Canadian Centre on Disability Studies, and the Public Health Agency of Canada. She has been published across a range of journals, including: *Journal of International Development, International Journal for Equity in Health, BMC Health Services Research, Women's Health and Urban Life,* and *Research Integrity and Peer Review.* Of note, Gemma authored a *Primer on Intersectional Qualitative Research* (2014) and co-developed an *Intersectionality-Based Policy Analysis Framework* (2012) that has been applied in various global sectors.

Nathan Lachowsky, PhD, is an Associate Professor in the School of Public Health and Social Policy at the University of Victoria in Australia and a Michael Smith Foundation for Health Research Scholar. He also serves as Research Director for the national Community-Based Research Centre Society (www.cbrc.net). Championing interdisciplinary and community-based approaches, he has conducted population health research with sexual and gender minoritized communities – particularly gay, bisexual, and queer men's communities – inclusive of Indigenous Two-Spirit, ethnoracialized, and trans and non-binary people across Canada and Aotearoa New Zealand. Nathan's research focuses on social and behavioral epidemiology and the importance of developing and analyzing mixed-methods data to inform public health practice, health service provision, interventions, and policy. He conducts interdisciplinary research within a social justice framework in order to achieve health equity for marginalized communities.

Malin Lindroth, PhD, has a PhD in Health and Society, and is a registered nurse specialized in school health nursing. She is an assistant professor in sexology and sexuality studies, and teaches at the master program in sexology at Malmö University in Sweden. Her research mainly concerns sexual health and rights for young people in secure state care, for transgender people, and also for people in homelessness as well as sexual and reproductive health and rights (SRHR) in higher education in Sweden. Ongoing projects involve rights-based sex education for young men in prisons. Recent publications include "Sexual and reproductive health and rights (SRHR) among young people in secure state care and their non-incarcerated peers – a qualitative, descriptive and comparative study" published in *European Journal of Social Work* (2020), and "On the outskirts of the charmed circle – challenges and limitations of sexual health promotion to young people in secure state care" published in *Sexuality Research and Social Policy* (2020).

Sizulu Moyo, MBChB, MPH, PhD, is a Research Director at the Human Sciences Research Council (HSRC) in South Africa. She has extensive public health and research experience and has led numerous multi-disciplinary research projects working with teams of local, national, and international stakeholders and collaborators on tuberculosis (TB) and HIV research projects and large-scale surveys. These projects include TB vaccine trials, the first South African national TB prevalence survey, the 5th South African national HIV survey, and the South African national COVID-19 prevalence survey. Dr. Moyo also has experience in health systems and programmatic research. Before joining the HSRC, she was an epidemiologist focusing on drug-resistant TB. She has also worked in the area of TB vaccine trials prior to which she was a practicing clinician. Her publication record spans the authoring and co-authoring of journal articles, conference presentations and research reports on TB and HIV.

Olanrewaju Oladimeji, PhD, is currently a visiting scholar at the Department of Global Health and Population, Harvard T.H. Chan School of Public Health, in Boston, Massachusetts, USA. He graduated with MBBS and MSc from the University of Ibadan, Nigeria. He completed his PhD in Public Health at the University of KwaZulu-Natal, South Africa. He has been involved in the implementation of large TB and HIV surveys in Sub-Saharan Africa countries. His publication record includes authoring and co-authoring several articles, and the impact of his research is reflected in a number of high-profile citations (Google Scholar: 13,941 and Web of Science: 13,291). His current h-index is 28 and i10-index is 39 (Google Scholar). He serves on the Editorial Board of several journals, including *PLoS One* and BMC journals. He has adjunct affiliations with universities and serves in various academic committees. He is a member of the National Young Academy in South Africa and Nigeria.

Nancy Poole, PhD, is the Director of the British Columbia Centre of Excellence for Women's Health in Vancouver, Canada, and the Prevention Lead for the CanFASD Research Network.

Priscilla Reddy, PhD, is the Strategic Lead at the Human Sciences Research Council and Research Associate at the Nelson Mandela University in South Africa. She is a specialist in behavioral science and health promotion research having obtained her PhD at Maastricht University in the Netherlands. She has extensive experience in research and intervention development in noncommunicable disease (NCD) and communicable disease, as well as implementation science and translational research. She served on the Institute of Medicine (IOM) Committee for the Evaluation of the President's Emergency Plan for AIDS Relief (PEPFAR); the IOM Committee: Scaling Up Treatment for the Global AIDS Pandemic – Challenges and Opportunities; Africa Tobacco Control Committee of the Network of African Science Academies (NASAC); and the National Academies. Her work in risk factors and determinants for NCDs over the past 25 years includes a socio-behavioral trial of smoking cessation and harm reduction, as well as three national surveys of youth risk behaviors.

Cara Tannenbaum, MD, MSc, is a Professor in the Faculties of Medicine and Pharmacy at the Université de Montréal in Canada. She was appointed Scientific Director of the Institute of Gender and Health for the Canadian Institutes of Health Research in 2015. In this capacity, Dr. Tannenbaum works with researchers and organizations nationally and internationally to catalyze policy and practice changes to increase representation of sex and gender from an intersectional perspective among those who conduct as well as those who benefit from scientific research. She boasts over 150 scientific publications, over 200 media engagements, and is the recipient of several awards including the May Cohen Gender Equity Award from the Association of Faculties of Medicine Canada and the Betty Havens Knowledge Transfer Award from the Canadian Institutes of Health Research.

Krystle van Hoof, MA, has held a variety of leadership positions within the not-for-profit sector, the federal government and the United Nations over the past two decades. She is currently the Managing Director and CEO of Healthy Brains, Healthy Lives, a large-scale neuroscience initiative at McGill University in Montreal, Quebec, Canada. Prior to this position, Krystle held the position of Assistant Director at the Institute of Gender and Health, one of 13 institutes that make up the Canadian Institutes of Health Research. An expert in strategic communications, Krystle has worked in private sector marketing as well as non-profit communications and has led communications departments for two national Canadian associations – work that has been recognized with national awards. Krystle has a Master's in Communication for Development from Malmö University in Sweden, a BA in Cultural Studies from York University in Canada, and a Professional Certificate in Knowledge Translation from the University of Toronto.

Fiona Warde, MD, completed her medical school training at Dalhousie University in Halifax, Nova Scotia, Canada, where she was actively involved in LGBTQ+ health research and the Student Diversity and Inclusion Committee. For her under-graduate research project, she completed a scoping review assessing the delivery of LGBTQ+ health topics in undergraduate medical curricula in Canada. In her role as co-chair, she assisted with creating curricular and policy changes relating to diversity and inclusion issues. As well, under her leadership the Dalhousie Medical Students' Society became active participants in the yearly Halifax Pride Parade. Fiona is now a first-year Medical Resident in the Department of Family Medicine at Queen's University in Kingston, Ontario, and intends to pursue a career in Family Medicine with a focus on care for LGBTQ+ elders.

Nompumelelo Zungu, PhD, is a Research Director at the Human Sciences Research Council in South Africa; an Associate Researcher at the University of Pretoria, Department of Psychology, in South Africa; and the Editor-in-Chief of the SAHARA Journal. She has a PhD in Psychology from the University of Cape Town, South Africa. She has expertise and special interest in the social aspects and social determinants of health, HIV, gender-based violence (GBV), mental health – specifically trauma and anxiety disorders, and risk and sexual behavior among men and adolescents. She has over 18 years of research experience and has been a principal investigator (PI), co-PI, and a chief of party on several national surveys and research projects on HIV and AIDS, health, and mental health. She is one of the PIs on the 1st South African National Gender-Based Violence Survey and the 6th National HIV Prevalence and Incidence Survey. She has co-authored over 51 journal articles, 9 book chapters, and 21 research reports.

Chapter 1
Introduction: Sex- and Gender-Based Analysis (SGBA) and Public Health

Jacqueline Gahagan and Mary K. Bryson

Canada is regarded as a global leader in seeking gender equity in mandating sex- and gender-based analysis (SGBA) in federal government initiatives, programmes and policies; and in continuing to advocate for the uptake of SGBA more broadly. However, there exists a longstanding differential in the uptake of SGBA in many fields, and public health is noted as a field that is lagging behind in the integration of SGBA. This book offers analyses of the intersection of SGBA in Canada and internationally in relation to the practice of public health with a focus on a number of core public health concerns such as HIV prevention, tobacco and alcohol use, cancer care, tuberculosis (TB), pandemics, and sexual health, among others. These topics continue to be highly relevant to the practice of public health in Canada as well as globally and are meant to offer the reader insights into a number of the current debates and discussions on the state of knowledge and action on SGBA in public health.

The Role of Public Health

At its core, the role of public health is to protect the aggregate of the health of populations. According to the World Health Organization (WHO), public health is defined as "… the art and science of preventing disease, prolonging life and promoting health through the organized efforts of society" (Committee of Inquiry into the Future Development of the Public Health Function, 1988). In the Canadian context,

J. Gahagan (✉)
Faculty of Health, Dalhousie University, Halifax, NS, Canada
e-mail: jgahagan@dal.ca

M. K. Bryson
Department of Language and Literacy Education, Faculty of Education, University of British Columbia, Vancouver, BC, Canada

© Springer Nature Switzerland AG 2021
J. Gahagan, M. K. Bryson (eds.), *Sex- and Gender-Based Analysis in Public Health*, https://doi.org/10.1007/978-3-030-71929-6_1

the Public Health Agency of Canada (PHAC) has a clear mandate to "promote and protect the health of Canadians through leadership, partnership, innovation and action in public health" (Government of Canada, 2020).

What is less clear is how these key mandates are enacted in relation to SGBA in the context of pressing public health issues that impact on the health of populations at the margins, such as those experiencing pandemics, addictions, and infectious and bloodborne diseases such as HIV, among others. The complex interplay between a variety of intersecting determinants of health, some modifiable and some non-modifiable, further compounds issues of poor health outcomes. While the focus of this book is on the impact of SGBA in public health, it is important to note that sex and gender cannot be understood in isolation from other determinants of health.

While SGBA ensures consideration is given to both sex (biological/physiological factors) and gender (sociocultural factors), concerns that matter to health outcomes, other intersecting issues such as age, race, socioeconomic status, education and access to health care also play a significant role in both the ways in which health can be negatively or positively impacted. Given this, the chapters in this book illustrate how and why both sex and gender and other determinants of health should be meaningfully addressed in the development of public health interventions, their implementation and their evaluation to further our understanding of what works, for whom and why. In this book, we trace relevant historical evolutions of SGBA and examine their applications to pressing public health issues. We also address why SGBA matters in advancing the health of women, men, girls and boys and gender-diverse populations. The overarching purpose of this book is to further our understanding of the links between SGBA and public health. Each of the following chapters offers a particular view of the utility of SGBA and offers concrete examples of SGBA in action in the realm of public health both nationally and internationally.

Part I: The SGBA Terrain

The first part of the book, "The SGBA Terrain", offers two chapters, both of which examine the issue of SGBA in public health, its application and its absence from more current debates about the ways in which public health interventions need to address in a more tailored fashion the unique needs of socially and economically marginalized segments of the population. These chapters underscore what is at stake in this book as a whole: the claim that rigorous public health research and interventions need to take both sex and gender into account in their explanatory models as well as the design of contexts for health care as well as health promotion. Both chapters in this part offer accounts of the complexities of SGBA as a mode of analysis of public health approaches that affords greater attention to models that allow us to explain health disparities and to detect the kinds of biases that prevent an accurate and evidence-informed mode of the analysis of population health diversity.

In Chap. 2, Shirin Heidari examines how sex and gender in public health are considered and addressed in different policies, strategies and approaches that guide and fund public health research, policy development and the design of public health programme interventions. Whereas public health research is typically framed in conceptual language and frameworks anchored in objectivity, Heidari's analysis distinguishes between large-scale institutional commitments to equity in public health research and settings and the actual cultural and material contexts wherein norms that guide decision-making concerning research funding, ethics review boards, publication and the design of large-scale interventions actually reflect narrow norms in relation to gender. Heidari's careful comparative reading of various national research funding organizations' requirements for applicants to identify the ways in which their proposed research takes gender into account provides clear evidence of the variability in institutional expectations concerning the value and the necessity of including a gender lens in the design of public health research.

The conceptual and practical problems for public health caused by the interchangeable use of sex and gender concepts in research and care settings and models are the subject of Natisha Dukhi, Priscilla Reddy and Nompumelelo Zungu's chapter on "Sex- and Gender-Based Analyses and Advancing Population Health." In Chap. 3, the authors make a compelling case for the greater integration of SGBA in advancing population health in order to address key drivers of poor health outcomes. The promotion of SGBA is ongoing in health and health outcome research. However, challenges exist in the research process with the continuous use of sex and gender concepts interchangeably. The authors argue that these concepts are not synonymous but rather intersect and are interrelated. There has been increased confusion in the contribution of both sex and gender to population health and health outcomes, leading to missed opportunities for the development of appropriate population health policies and interventions. In this chapter, the authors argue that the core elements of SGBA are not just limited to the concepts of sex and gender but also include key issues of diversity and equity. Within a population, diversity refers to the observable variations such as ethnicity and age distinctions and the not-so-evident differences such as spiritual or religious persuasion and sexual orientation. Dukhi, Reddy and Zungu's chapter concludes by sketching out an ideal setting wherein women, men and gender-diverse populations would have the right to health, including access to health services tailored for more equitable health outcomes in the face of systemic disparities in population health. For these authors, SGBA is a progressive development in population health in the fact that it not only is inclusive of the individuals affected or involved but also is important in addressing the gaps in research, literature, policy and data. To address key population health issues, the authors argue that research data must identify the strengths and limitations related to the core concepts of SGBA, as this may influence health status, health intervention development and implementation, policy address, delivery of health services and, overall, health research.

Part II: SGBA Matters

Part II of this book, "SGBA Matters", includes chapters that focus more explicitly on SGBA viewed through the lens of more specific public health content issues including HIV and AIDS, tobacco use, cancer, alcohol use, tuberculosis, sexual health and pandemics. The chapters in this part review current debates on the key tensions in integrating SGBA approaches into public health interventions across a very wide range of practical public health domains.

In "HIV prevention", Jacqueline Gahagan and Shari L. Dworkin examine the issues associated with the early epidemiology of HIV in North America and the AIDS risk paradigms or vulnerability paradigms and how these have served to overlook populations of cisgender and transgender women and heterosexual men in public health responses. In Chap. 4, the authors argue that notions of HIV sexual risk-taking and the overarching absence of heterosexually identified cisgender and transgender women and heterosexual men from early HIV public health interventions and clinical trials served to further the narrative whereby HIV risk-taking was regarded as a stereotypically male characteristic and that, as a consequence, other populations were not seen to be at risk. The authors proceed to underscore the ways in which the use of the terms "sex" and "gender" interchangeably in HIV-related public health and clinical interventions was and continues to be problematic in understanding both the physiological and gendered interplay contributing to HIV infection. For example, the use of single-sex, cisgender male-only HIV clinical trial data to determine HIV RNA levels as the de facto measure for the initiation of anti-retroviral therapy (ART), and the subsequent extrapolation of pharmacokinetics and effectiveness data on ART to cisgender women, was problematic. Further, the lack of reference to and framing of the gender-related social determinants contributing to differential HIV infection rates, access to and uptake of HIV testing, treatment, access to and use of pre-exposure prophylaxis (PrEP) and issues of disclosure, among others, served to limit our understanding of the pandemic among other diverse populations. Chapter 4 concludes with a discussion on the need for gender-transformative approaches to HIV prevention, treatment and support in public health, particularly in relation to addressing the enduring disparities in access to and uptake of public health interventions aimed at reducing the burden of HIV in the North American context.

For Lorraine Greaves and Natalie Hemsing, SGBA offers a very integral lens for the analysis of health disparities related to tobacco use. Chapter 5 provides a review of the public health problems related to tobacco use, which is a key public health issue globally and the leading cause of preventable death in the world with over seven million deaths per year and leading to one billion deaths in this century. The authors of Chap. 5 provide a careful review of the gendered patterns of tobacco use, with more men than women using tobacco and often starting and quitting first. Ending tobacco use is the subject of the world's first and only public health treaty, the World Health Organization Framework Convention on Tobacco Control, with 168 signatories worldwide. While the tobacco industry has consistently applied a sex- and gender-based analysis to tobacco in production, advertising and marketing, public health has failed to integrate sex and gender into its prevention and cessation responses. Feminist writers have critiqued the generic "one-size-fits-all" public health approach for several decades, arguing for more tailored, equitable and gendered responses. In the face of spreading cigarette use in low-income countries, continuing smoking among vulnerable populations in high-income countries and new e-cigarette products generating dependence among users, Greaves and Hemsing conclude by claiming that the call for a tailored sex- and gender-based analysis to tobacco control, which has gender and health equity as its ultimate goal, is even more important and urgent.

Jacqueline Gahagan, Mary Bryson and Fiona Warde's chapter, "Beyond 'Women's Cancers': Sex and Gender in Cancer Health and Care", explores and contests the male/female binary that historically and into the present day organizes public health models and concepts pertaining to cancer health risk, diagnoses and care. The authors report on "Cancer's Margins" (http://www.lgbtcancer.ca), Canada's first nationally funded, nationwide project to investigate experiences of breast and/or gynaecologic cancer health through a SGBA lens with a specific focus on sexual and/or gender marginalities. In Chap. 6, the authors describe their findings based on a qualitative analysis of LGBQ/T2 cancer patient narratives and report how it is that sexual and/or gender minority cancer patients punctuate the otherwise lockstep assemblage of their cancer treatment decision-making with persistent attempts to resist, thwart and otherwise manage the possibility of discrimination and, likewise, the probability of institutional erasure in care settings. The authors state that the Cancer's Margins project findings illustrate the value added to the body of research on gender, sexuality and cancer, by means of the application of an SGBA lens to an area of significant importance to the domain of public health.

The problems posed to public health research and care by the failure to disaggregate concepts and related bodies of data by gender, that other authors have outlined, are the focus of Chap. 7, "Tuberculosis and the Relevance of Sex- and Gender-Based Analysis". Sizulu Moyo, Olanrewaju Oladimeji, Jeremiah Chikovore and Nompulelelo Zungu outline how population groups that are at greater risk of TB are often also at higher risk for health disparities. Evidence consistently shows that the burden of TB differs by sex, gender, poverty and other determinants of health. In fact, TB notification and prevalence survey data have shown a higher burden of TB in men than in women globally. The authors make a persuasive case for how it is that gender norms and roles influence and are influenced by a variety of determinants of health, including sociodemographic, behavioural and economic factors, which, in turn, influence the risk of acquisition of *Mycobacterium tuberculosis bacilli* and of developing active TB, as well as the response to the disease at local, community and national levels. Their chapter documents how it is that while TB data are generally disaggregated by sex, the disaggregation tends to be broad and masks differences within groups by age and other important factors. Understanding and reporting TB with a consideration of these factors is critical to ensure equity in addressing the TB disease burden with appropriate strategies. There remains a need for detailed SGBA of TB interventions at various levels and within local contexts in order to inform strategies that will be effective in supporting the public health goal of ending TB by 2035.

Following Moyo, Oladimeji, Chikovore and Zungu's discussion of the benefits of SBGA in shedding light on population complexities relative to TB, Nancy Poole's analysis of gender in relation to girl's and women's alcohol use provides a great deal of evidence of the possible benefits to public health and of the application of a gender lens to better document and address a major area of health disparities. In Chap. 8, Nancy Poole provides a convincing case for the argument that gender-based health disparities in the area of public health research concerning alcohol demonstrate and support the acute need for sex, gender and intersectional analysis to be brought to bear on the topic of women and alcohol, the uptake to date by public health and much needed directions forward. Poole's cogent SGBA in the area of alcohol use and health disparities stresses the profound consequences of the failure to take gender into account in public health and how this inaction has parallels from the eighteenth century on. Poole concludes with a call to action on public health models that offer gendered, health-promoting and harm-reducing approaches.

In Chap. 9, "Sexual Health Promotion", Allison Carter, Nathan Lachowsky and Jacqueline Gahagan review evidence on SGBA and global initiatives pertaining to sexual health promotion. The authors argue that operationalizing an SGBA-informed approach to sexual health promotion is crucial to our understanding of how differently situated individuals and populations experience sexuality, which entails not just freedom from sexual risk and harm (e.g. STBBI, unplanned pregnancies and gender-based violence) but also the right to sexual autonomy and well-being in its broadest sense (e.g. desires, identities, experiences and relationships). The authors' careful analysis provides a compelling overview of research that points to how it is that the absence of holistic conceptualizations of sexual health promotion and SGBA in all aspects of the science, philosophy and practice of public health—historically and in the present day—means that significant knowledge, education and programming gaps continue to exist with respect to sexual health on a global scale.

Olena Hankivsky provides a very timely analysis of the value of an SGBA approach to research and public health interventions regarding pandemics. Hankivsky argues that understandings of the differential impacts of pandemics on men, women, boys and girls of diverse backgrounds have been hampered by the relative lack of attention to the *interplay* of complex factors and influencing forces that underpin pandemics, including but not limited to gender. Specifically, what is needed is a more sophisticated and transformative analysis. Chapter 10, "Understanding Pandemics Through a Sex- and Gender-Based Analysis Plus (SGBA+) Lens", explores the potential of an intersectional mode of SGBA to advance our knowledge of the differential impacts of pandemics. A major contribution of Hankivsky's research is to examine and integrate what intersectionality requires of SGBA and the implications for worldwide public health crises that have threatened the global community, such as severe acute respiratory syndrome (SARS), Ebola, Zika and most recently COVID-19. Through an examination of these examples, she illustrates what has been emphasized and what is often missing in the analysis of public health emergencies and pandemics. Hankivsky also demonstrates the value added of an intersectionality multilevel, power-focused analysis of interacting factors, processes and structures for generating better evidence to advance understandings and responses to pandemics.

Part III: The Responsibilities of Public Health

In the final part of this book, "The Responsibilities of Public Health", the authors explore the implications of SGBA and public health in the areas of the social determinants of health for incarcerated young people, gender-transformative approaches in public health and, finally, translation, implementation and engagement in public health.

This final part offers three chapters that address the way forward with SGBA in public health. While some progress has been made in adding sex-specific and/or gender-relevant considerations to major public health issues, further work is needed in ensuring the next generation of public health practitioners has sufficient fluency in SGBA to allow for the meaningful and measurable indicators of success to be incorporated into various public health interventions. Without such intentional uptake and integration of SGBA from within the discipline and practice of public health (and beyond), we will continue to see the health disparities among males, females and gender-diverse populations in relation to the significant public health issues as illustrated in the core content areas of this book. Despite Canada being regarded as a leader in SGBA, moving towards a purposeful adoption of SGBA within public health nationally and globally will require leadership and innovation on the part of public health trainees as they take up decision-making roles within various aspects of their public health practice in partnership with their colleagues in critical social science and beyond.

In Malin Lindroth and Catrine Andersson's chapter, "Sex- Gender-Based Analysis and the Social Determinants of Health: Public Health, Human Rights and Incarcerated Youth", the authors examine the context of young people incarcerated in secure state care institutions in Sweden to illustrate how SGBA is key to public health responses for incarcerated populations. Specifically, they describe how incarcerated young people experience interconnected and negative health outcomes related to a variety of social determinants of health prior to their incarceration, which are further exacerbated as a consequence of incarceration. The major contributions of this informative intersectional research on gender, sexual health and human rights are that the data cited by the authors, and their data analysis, provide compelling evidence concerning the varied and major impacts of a lack of access to sexual health promotion tailored with an SGBA lens, including a lack of preventive and promoting public health measures informed by a human rights perspective within secure care institutions.

In Chap. 12, "Gender-Transformative Public Health Approaches", Olena Hankivsky and Gemma Hunting provide a detailed and compelling account of the more complex and dynamic modes of carrying out an SGBA analysis in health research and/or the design of care models in public health by drawing on two major threads of research to date in this area: intersectionality and gender-transformative approaches. The authors' intersectional mode of SGBA contests single-variable modes of the analysis of gender as a social determinant of health. The authors provide a wide array of evidence that supports the argument that gender is never a standalone factor or cause of inequity. Gender interacts with other factors and determinants such as age, disability, socioeconomic status and geography to shape experiences, life chances and health across different groups of women, men and gender-diverse populations. Hankivsky and Hunting take up current work that documents the growing acknowledgement of the importance of an intersectional approach to SGBA and gives us occasion to reflect on how intersectionality is transforming the entire landscape of public health, including the development and strengthening of mainstream frameworks and tools such as gender-transformative approaches (GTA). Finally, the authors provide GTA examples that mention or integrate intersectionality and the development, in the Canadian context, of sex- and gender-based analysis plus (SGBA+), which is an explicit attempt to integrate intersectionality.

In the final chapter, Krystal van Hoof and Cara Tannenbaum, in "Translation, Implementation and Engagement", take into account the significance of an intersectional approach to knowledge translation as understood through the lens of SGBA. In Chap. 13, the authors explore the argument that ensuring public health policies and programmes are evidence-informed and equitable and requires the appropriate consideration of sex and gender, along with other intersecting social determinants of health (e.g. age, race, ethnicity, socioeconomic status). Van Hoof and Tannenbaum argue that sex and gender must, therefore, be accounted for in both the content of the evidence used to inform public health and the processes by which stakeholders are engaged to translate and implement the evidence through policies and programmes. The authors demonstrate how it is that even without sex and gender considerations, it has been a long-standing challenge to transfer high-quality, timely and relevant research knowledge into policy and practice across all domains of health and medicine. Accordingly, thoughtful and purposeful reflection and planning are warranted to maximize the potential positive impacts of SGBA in public health.

References

Committee of Inquiry into the Future Development of the Public Health Function. (1988). *Public health in England: Report of the Committee of Inquiry into the Future Development of the Public Health Function (Cm. 289)*. London: The Stationery Office.
Government of Canada. (2020). *About the Public Health Agency of Canada*. https://www.canada. ca/en/public-health/corporate/mandate/about-agency.html. Accessed 11 Dec 2020.

Part I
The SGBA Terrain

Chapter 2
Missing in Action: Sex- and Gender-Based Analysis (SGBA) in Public Health

Shirin Heidari

Public health strategies have been implemented over centuries to control and prevent disease and outbreaks and promote health. The World Health Organization (WHO) defines health in its constitution as "a state of complete physical, mental and social well-being and not merely the absence of disease or infirmity", and notes that public health aims to provide "maximum benefit for the largest number of people" and is rooted in principles of social justice. The right to health is a human right. The right to health is intrinsically linked to other rights (WHO, 2008a). "[H]ealth inequities arise from the societal conditions in which people are born, grow, live, work and age, referred to as social determinants of health" (Rio Political Declaration on Social Determinants of Health, 2011). The Committee on Economic, Social and Cultural Rights articulates that the right to health is an inclusive right, which includes among others the right to safe drinking water and adequate sanitation, safe food, adequate nutrition and housing, healthy working and environmental conditions, health-related education and information and gender equality (WHO, 2008a).

Gender inequality and gender power relations constitute a critical determinant of health, which operates at micro, meso and macro levels. The most recent COVID-19 pandemic reveals this reality (Wenham et al., 2020; Heidari et al. 2020). Intersecting with other social markers of inequality, including but not limited to age, race, ethnicity, sexual orientation, gender identity or expression, disability and migration status, gender shapes the conditions and circumstances in which people live, work, play, love and age and creates differential experiences of illness and wellness (Sen et al., 2007; Hankivsky, 2012; UNFPA, 2020). As such, disregarding gender

S. Heidari (✉)
GENDRO, Geneva, Switzerland

Global Health Centre, Graduate Institute of International and Development Studies, Geneva, Switzerland
e-mail: s.heidari@gendro.org

© Springer Nature Switzerland AG 2021
J. Gahagan, M. K. Bryson (eds.), *Sex- and Gender-Based Analysis in Public Health*, https://doi.org/10.1007/978-3-030-71929-6_2

dynamics in public health can undermine the fundamental principles of social justice and the right to highest attainable standard of health (Heidari & Doyle, 2020).

Yet, gender blindness and gender bias in public health is ubiquitous. Gender bias in public health is based on the flawed assumption that women's, men's and transgender and gender-non-conforming individuals' health situations, risks and experiences are similar. Knowledge about one, in this approach, can be extrapolated to the others. In reality, this is far from the truth. The historic androcentrism in public health research has resulted in a fragmented and partial understanding of sex- and gender-related differences and underlying causes for these differential heath experiences, social inequities and health outcomes, with a particularly egregious example constituted by the frequent omission of the experiences of women, transgender and gender-non-conforming people.

In recent years, we have seen a rapid amplification of publications, statements and initiatives generating evidence and raising concerns about the entrenched gender bias in research and reporting in health sciences, particularly in the field of medicine and public health, as one of the main reasons for observed gender disparities and inequities in health (Nature, 2010; Heidari & Bachelet, 2018; Clayton & Collins, 2014; JAMA 2003; Gahagan et al., 2015; Purnell et al., 2005). This advocacy has resulted in a growing awareness about the complex interaction of sex and gender and its intersection with other determinants of health, the differential health outcomes and healthcare experiences at all stages of life and across the globe. This awareness has resulted in the proliferation of sex and gender-responsive approaches in public health research, policies and programmes.

An important milestone has been the high-level recognition of the importance of gender as a critical determinant of health. In 2008, the 60th World Health Assembly adopted resolution 60.25, which is the WHO's first (and to date the only) gender strategy (WHO, 2008b). The strategy urges "[m]ember States to formulate national strategies for addressing gender issues in health policies, programs, research, and planning processes" and calls on them "to ensure that a gender-equality perspective is incorporated in all levels of health-care delivery and services" (WHO, 2008b).

In the same year, global ministerial research for health, development and equity launched the Bamako Call to Action on research for health, in which they state, "[T]he global research for health agenda should be determined by national and regional agendas and priorities, with due attention to gender and equity consideration" (The Lancet 2008; World Health Organization 2008). The Sustainable Development Goals (SDGs) further highlight the importance of sex disaggregated data. The global SDG indicator framework adopted to track progress has as its overarching principle that "indicators should be disaggregated, where relevant, by income, sex, age, race, ethnicity, migratory status, disability and geographic location, or other characteristics" (United Nations General Assembly 2014). The high-level recognition of gender as an important determinant of health, while insufficient to transform the public health research system and culture, is certainly a giant step in the right direction and indication of notable advancements.

In this chapter, I examine how sex and gender in public health are considered and addressed in different strategies that guide, fund and oversee public health research, policies and practices. The intention of this chapter is to highlight some areas of notable progress and to identify where actions are still missing.

Public Health Research

Public health research has an enormous value for society. In addition to improving individual health and well-being, public health research has a significant impact on advancing population health, increasing life expectancy and productivity and contributing to social and economic development. Through public health and medical research, we are able to advance our understanding of diseases and risk factors, understand transmission patterns, discover new prevention modalities or therapeutic interventions or improve existing approaches and identify ways to improve delivery of public health interventions. New knowledge informs future research hypotheses and directions and contributes to optimizing models of care. Further, public health research informs normative guidelines and health policies, influences prioritization and regulation of interventions and shapes how we organize health systems, manage health expenses and effectively deliver health services (Tulchinsky et al., 2015; Schneider, 2012).

Public health policies and practices are committed ethically and institutionally to be grounded in and informed by the best scientific knowledge and high quality and reliable evidence, "conscious of the need to address the social determinants of health, including those related to gender, income, education, ability, conflict and ethnicity" (Ministerial Summit on Health Research 2004). The World Health Assembly (WHA), the highest governing body of the World Health Organization, in resolution 58.34 acknowledges, "High-quality research and the generation and application of knowledge are critical for achieving the internationally agreed health-related development goals, including those contained in the United Nations Millennium Declaration, improving the performance of health systems, advancing human development, and attaining equity in health" (WHO, 2005). Mobilization in support of global development goals further underlines the need for sound ethical research in the realization of the Sustainable Development Goals, including the aspiration of Universal Health Coverage by 2030 (Scientific Advisory Board of the UN Secretary-General, 2016; United Nations, 2017). Hence, improvements in health are dependent on robust ethical research that promises the greatest potential to address health inequities. As such, the generation of gender-sensitive evidence is critical to address health inequities originating from rigid gender norms and roles and unequal gender power relations.

Health research has historically been a male endeavour and based on white, cis-gender, heterosexual male experience. Androcentrism in health and medical research is being increasingly questioned and debated. Growing evidence shows how women are underrepresented in clinical trials, experiences of women and gender-non-conforming persons are overlooked in health research and data analysis fails to examine sex differences and gender dynamics (Palmer-Ross et al., 2021 Curno et al., 2016; Sherman et al., 1995; Holdcroft, 2007; Ramasubbu et al., 2001; Schiebinger, 2003; Morselli et al., 2016; Davis, 2017; Winter et al., 2016; Reisner et al., 2016). While initial advocacy efforts were intended to expose the disadvantages that women face as a result of this androcentric approach, there is an emerging discourse that underscores that the benefits of gender-sensitive research accrue also for men and gender-non-confirming people. Research into notions of traditional and hegemonic masculinity shows how rigid gender norms and expectations can result in greater premature mortality or barriers to health care and foregone health needs among men, including those of diverse sexual orientation and gender identity. Addressing gender bias in research, therefore, requires that both sex and gender, and their intersection with other critical variables such as age, race and ethnicity, sexual orientation, gender identity and expression and disability, are integral parts of research design, considered in data collection and systematically taken into account throughout the research process, including in relation to data analysis, reporting and knowledge translation.

Research is conducted within an ecosystem of complex social institutions, and the process of change is both challenging and slow. The prime purpose of research is to advance knowledge over time through scientific objectivity, conceptual innovation and excellence. The health research ecosystem consists of a number of checkpoints, operated through gatekeeping functions to safeguard research integrity and foster excellence. These functions are carried out by peers, who evaluate the soundness, quality and excellence of research and shape what constitutes knowledge and evidence (Merton, 1973). Funding agencies decide what research to fund, and thereby shape the knowledge that is produced. Research can be conducted only when approved by ethics committees responsible for ensuring that research, particularly involving human participants, respects core ethical principles. Academic journals constitute another critical gatekeeping function in this ecosystem, as research findings become "knowledge" only when they have successfully undergone rigorous peer-evaluation, been scrutinized by editors and enter the public domain in the form of academic articles published in scholarly journals. Together, these gatekeepers define the standards and criteria for quality and ethical research, and thereby, shape the construction of excellence.

Despite the growing recognition of the importance of sex and gender in research as key to quality, reproducibility and soundness, their relevance is rarely evaluated at different stages of the research process, or if considered, often only narrowly limited to concern for the "vulnerability" of pregnant and breastfeeding women.

Many of these gatekeeping functions, historically have and to a large extent still today, are occupied by men, who, in the academic evaluation of funding proposals, research protocols or scientific manuscripts, determine and deploy a narrow framework for the identification of "merit" and "excellence". Through this process, perhaps subconsciously, they reproduce gender inequalities and implicitly legitimize gender-blind approaches to research in the research proposals they fund, study protocols they approve and material they publish. The research system has been said to be "riddled with prejudice", sexism and nepotism (Wenneras & Wold, 1997).

Gatekeepers in research can be important catalysts for change and can accelerate the systematic integration of sex and gender dimensions and meaningful gender analysis, and improve integrated reporting across research eco-systems.

Research Funding Agencies

Health research funding agencies play a pivotal role, as they are one of the primary gatekeepers with the ability to influence research design and encourage investigators to formulate research questions in ways that correctly and appropriately capture various sex and gender dimensions. This consideration at the design stage is critical to guide sample size calculation, recruitment strategies, appropriate data collection, and in turn meaningful sub-group and intersectional gender analysis. Several research funding agencies have come to acknowledge the importance of sex and gender in their funding programmes (Clayton & Collins, 2014; CIHR Institute on Gender and Health, 2018; Helsinki Group on Gender in Research and Innovation Position, 2017). Some national funding agencies have introduced policies to encourage and even mandate gender-sensitive research (European Commission, 2009). There are great variations in the formulation and implementation of these policies and only a few, if any, *require* sex and gender considerations as a condition for receiving funding (Clayton & Collins, 2014; Hankivsky et al., 2018; European Commission, 2020).

One of the first agencies to introduce such a policy was the US National Institutes of Health (NIH). In 1993, in response to women's health advocacy, the US Congress passed the NIH Revitalization Act, mandating the inclusion of women and minorities in clinical research and examination of differences with a greater emphasis on sex-based differences between men and women (National Institutes of Health, 1993). This policy applies to all NIH-supported biomedical and behavioural research involving human subjects and is the first to state that any "any grant, cooperative agreement or contract" and other support will not be awarded if it does not comply with this policy. It further requires awardees to annually report on "enrollment of women and men, and the race and ethnicity of research participants" (National Institutes of Health, 1993). In 2014, NIH announced that it will complement its current policy by requiring that research funding applicants also "report their plans for the balance of male and female cells and animals in preclinical studies [...] with parallel changes in review activities and requirements" (Clayton & Collins, 2014).

Nevertheless, there is evidence of inadequate compliance with the NIH guidelines despite the mandatory requirements. In a 2011 review of phase III clinical trial eligible for enrolment by both men and women funded by NIH between 1995 and 2010, authors report that only 37% of trial participants were women. Only 28% of published articles reporting the findings of these trials mentioned sex and/or gender in the results, with only a third providing a sub-group analysis (Foulkes, 2011). This is in line with the systematic review of HIV clinical trials between 1994 and 2011 by Curno et al. in 2016 who also reported that trials with antiretrovirals (ARV) that were fully or partially funded by NIH "included a significantly lower proportion of women compared with studies funded by other sources, indicating that the US federal regulations have limited impact on the inclusion of women in ARV clinical trials" (Curno et al., 2016).

The Canadian government introduced a similar policy, Health Canada's "Gender-Based Analysis Policy", in 2000 (Government of Canada, 2000). This policy was replaced in 2009 by Health Portfolio's "Sex and Gender-Based Analysis Policy", which highlights "that biological, economic and social differences between women and men contribute to differences in health risks, health services use, health system interaction and health outcomes" (Government of Canada, 2009). The Canadian Institutes of Health Research (CIHR) introduced guidelines in 2016 that support the implementation of the federal policy and encouraging integration of gender and sex-based analysis in health research (Canadian Institutes of Health Research 2016). Unlike the NIH Revitalization Act, the CIHR policy does require inclusion of specific groups. The CIHR requires applicants to answer specific questions on if and how sex and gender have been considered in their research protocol. These dimensions are also assessed by evaluators and reviewers and taken into account into the overall score. A review of funded applicants in the first year of the policy suggests an increase in affirmative responses to these questions (Johnson et al., 2014).

The European Commission has also been very proactive in articulating a cross-cutting gender policy for improving sex and gender considerations in the research it funds and underlines the importance of this approach and its added value in terms of gender equality, research excellence, innovation and business opportunities. In its flagship programme, Horizon 2020, the EU has dedicated funds to improve gender equality in research performing organizations, including gender mainstreaming in research content. One of the three objectives of gender equality in Horizon 2020 is "[i]ntegrating the gender dimension in research and innovation content" (European Commission, 2015). The European Institute for Gender Equality (EIGE) is another effort by the EU to advance gender equality in academia and gender mainstreaming in research content (EIGE 2015).

A comprehensive review of 45 key funding agencies across 36 countries by Hankivsky and colleagues provides an overview of gender policies in national research funding agencies and shows that 15 funding agencies, all of which are located in high-income countries, *mention* consideration of sex and gender in the content of research (Hankivsky et al., 2018). However, only a handful of the countries have incorporated requirements to integrate sex and gender dimensions in research grant application systems and offer practical guidance regarding the assessment of gender dimensions in research funding proposals.

The slowly growing number of gender-related requirements and policies in health research funding mechanisms indicates significant progress. However, there remains great variation in the effective implementation of these funding policies, and uptake across different disciplines. Having more (sex- and) gender-balanced research studies does not necessarily mean that the right data are collected or that data are analysed for capturing sex differences or identifying relevant gender dimensions. Neither does it mean that data are routinely reported disaggregated by sex. Furthermore, even mandatory requirements to report sex and gender dimensions in research funding proposals do not seem to be systematically assessed by reviewers or be reflected in the scores (Hankivsky et al., 2018). Moreover, an intersectional approach is rarely applied; policies do not adequately recognize the need to consider the intersection of gender with other health determinants such as sexual orientation, gender identity and expression, age, race or ethnicity, socio-economic status, refugee status and disability.

Research Ethics Committees

Research ethics committees (Ethics or Institutional Review Boards) constitute another critical gatekeeper in the research ecosystem. In almost all countries, prior ethical approval by an ethics committee is required to conduct research with human or animal subjects. Research ethics committees (RECs) are tasked with reviewing proposed research protocols with human or animal subjects in order to confirm that they comply with international and local ethical standards. RECs can approve, ask for modifications or reject research proposals on ethical grounds and have the authority to stop a research project if is deemed to violate core ethical principles. Academic journals can also refuse publication of research that does not provide proof of ethical approval by a legitimate review board. RECs hold incredible power and authority to allow what research can or cannot be conducted.

The ethical concerns in health research related to gender have historically been limited to exclusions of pregnant women or women of childbearing potential due to the potential harm of experimental interventions on the foetus, often disregarding implications of such exclusion or the likelihood of potential risks in case of participation (National Research Act 1974). This policy has effectively led to exclusions of women of reproductive age from clinical studies. However, the validity of such a categorical exclusion has been contested (Kim et al., 2010). Inclusion of women in clinical studies is nowadays a requirement mandated by funding agencies, as indicated in the previous section. Ensuring informed choices of women and access to reproductive options, including contraception and safe abortion care, continues to be an important ethical rationale in clinical research (Committee on Ethical and Legal Issues Relating to the Inclusion of Women in Clinical Studies 1994). Exclusion of pregnant women in research is a topic of continued debate (Lyerly et al., 2008; Mastroianni et al., 1994; Van der Graaf et al., 2018). Participation of pregnant women in research is crucial to generate sufficient evidence about the safety and efficacy of interventions to address health concerns during pregnancy. This was particularly evident in the context of the Zika outbreak. Efforts are being made to address these shortcomings. For example, the United States Department of Health and Human Services has created a Task Force on Research Specific to Pregnant Women and Lactating Women (PRGLAC) to "address gaps in knowledge and research about safe and effective therapies for use during pregnancy and lactating women, and to explore ethical issues of including pregnant women and lactating women in clinical research" (NICHD 2018).

The gender aspects of ethical research extend beyond both female reproduction and the gender binary. Ethical concerns of gender bias in research are relevant to the principles of beneficence, i.e. doing good or maximizing the potential benefit; non-maleficence, i.e. doing no harm; and justice and equity, i.e. access to equitable, impartial, unbiased research (Lawrence & Rieder, 2007). Gender-biased research resulting in misleading findings can be harmful and, hence, should be a matter of ethical concern. The principle of justice also applies if the burden of disease falls on both men and women, and transgender or gender-non-conforming people, but the study population consists disproportionately of individuals of one sex or gender. "Access to [benefits of] research, not just protection from its risks, is a constitutive part of the ethical mandates governing clinical research" (Lyerly et al., 2008).

In certain health areas, such as HIV, there have been well-founded dedicated efforts on the ethical consideration of research with people with diverse sexual orientation and/or gender identity and expression, or particularly vulnerable populations, such as indigenous, racial or ethnic minorities, or people living with disabilities. However, in general, the needs and perspectives of people with diverse sexual orientation and gender identity or expression are often overlooked in public health research, including in areas where they experience greater burden of disease (Davis, 2017; Mayer et al., 2008; Alzahrani et al., 2019; The Lancet 2013; Adams et al., 2017; Baptiste-Roberts et al., 2017).

Academic Publishing

Poor and insufficient reporting of sex-disaggregated data and a lack of gender analysis remains one of the most persistent challenges in research. In the past decade, there has been an amplification of reviews, studies and commentaries that have generated evidence and shed light on persistent gender biases in reporting. Palmer-Ross et al. 2021; Avery and Clark 2016; Foulkes 2011b; Gahagan et al. 2015; S. Heidari and Bachelet 2018; Shirin Heidari et al. 2011, 2012; Rásky et al. 2017; Schiebinger et al. 2016; Welch et al. 2017; Wizemann 2012. According to the EU, between 2013 and 2017, only 1.79% of all publications within the 28 EU countries included a sex or gender dimension in reporting findings (Directorate-General for Research and Innovation 2019).

In 2012, the European Association of Science Editors established a Gender Policy Committee, and following a consultative process, published the Sex and Gender Equity in Research (SAGER) Guidelines in 2016 (Heidari et al., 2016). The publication of the SAGER guidelines was an effort to convene stakeholders and provide an ethical and scientific rationale for reporting of data disaggregated by sex, as a minimum, and the reporting of gender analysis, when appropriate, as a matter of routine. The SAGER guidelines offer a uniform set of criteria to support journal editors, peer reviewers and authors and facilitate a more systematic approach to gender-sensitive scholarly publication and communication (Heidari et al., 2016).

The guidelines also recommend practical steps for journal editors to operationalize the recommendations.

Journal editors are critical gatekeepers of science and have historically been instrumental in shaping research standards. Numerous reporting guidelines have been developed to address identified gaps and deficiencies, such as improving the transparency and complete reporting of randomized clinical trials (e.g. CONSORT) or systematic reviews (PRISMA). However, almost none of these reporting guidelines include reporting of sex and gender as a requirement that must be included in reporting. As such, the SAGER guidelines are meant to complement the existing guidelines, but ideally, sex and gender dimensions should be an integral and mandatory reporting component in all other reporting guidelines already required by most high-impact journals.

Increasingly, journals have been responding to these calls. Some high-impact journals and some publishers have adopted the SAGER guidelines and made public commitments to address the gender gap (refer Additional Resources section). There has yet to be an evaluation to assess to what extent these well-intended policies, such as SAGER guidelines, translate into active and routine enforcement and impact publication outcomes. Additional initiatives are required to ensure that these policies are accompanied by capacity building of editorial staff and training of peer reviewers.

Public Health Policies and Practices

Public health policies are meant to deal with a plethora of health risks, threats and demands of the population they serve. They need to manage and respond to a range of old and new public health concerns, from pandemics such as influenza, HIV and COVID-19 and outbreaks such as Zika and Ebola to the threat of antibiotic resistance to the growing burden of chronic diseases – cancer, cardiovascular diseases or mental health, to other widespread health concerns such as violence and gender-based violence – each area requires specific or different policy and programmatic strategies. Health promotion and fostering healthy lifestyles throughout life course, such as combating tobacco use, excessive alcohol consumption, promoting physical activity and reducing risk of injuries and violence, or planning to deal with the public health implications of climate change and natural disasters or conflicts, wars and other humanitarian crises also require strategic public health approaches. The successful implementation of these policies and strategies to meet the health needs of all persons equitably requires functional public health systems, thoughtful planning of human resources for health, equitable health insurance and social protection schemes and an enabling policy and legal environment with formal human rights provisions.

Sex and, to a greater extent, gender, function in intersection with other social markers to influence access to health information, exposure and propensity to risk and illness, prevalence and experience of disease and injuries, access to and utilization of health services, compliance with treatment and prevention recommendations and interaction with healthcare providers at health facilities. The organization and operation of public health systems, the location and timing of services and the working environment, capacity and attitudes of healthcare providers (and how patients are received, treated and by whom) can all facilitate or impede access to services and retention in care (Sen et al., 2007; Weber et al., 2019; Witter et al., 2017; Horton, 2019; George et al., 2019). Disrespect, abuse and violence against people of diverse sexual orientation, gender identity and expression as well as women in healthcare settings showcase how these discriminatory practices create impediments to equal and equitable access to services and quality care (Sen et al., 2018a; Matthen et al., 2018; Gonzales et al., 2016; Sen et al., 2018b; Human Rights Watch 2018). Preference, availability, mobility and quality of care are all shaped by gender norms, expectations and gender (in)equalities. Lack of basic health knowledge among healthcare providers about the basic health needs and concerns of gender-diverse populations is another example of the barriers within health systems (Mayer et al., 2008; Colpitts & Gahagan, 2016; Gahagan & Colpitts, 2017; Taylor & Bryson, 2016).

To illustrate how applying a gender lens can transform the public health response, one can turn to the experiences gained from the HIV field, which pioneered gender-responsive public health thinking. For example, the "feminization" of the HIV epidemic in Sub-Saharan Africa exposed the futility of the extensively sponsored ABC campaign – promoting abstinence, "being faithful" and condom use – among monogamous married women or women in partnership who were unable to remain abstinent or negotiate condom use, yet remained at high risk of HIV acquisition from their male partners. Understanding these dimensions led to innovation towards the development of female-controlled prevention modalities, such as microbicides, pre-exposure prophylaxis and dual protection from both HIV and unwanted pregnancy. Similarly, through gender-conscious research taking into account intersecting factors, public health professionals and activists could provide evidence of how sexual and gender-based violence impact women and girls, but also impact men who have sex with men and transgender populations, which represent groups that remain largely affected by HIV.

The current COVID-19 pandemic has once again exposed the fundamental influence of gender and its intersection with age, race and ethnicity, migration status, sexual orientation and gender identity on incidence, disease outcome and the experience of disease, the pandemic and the measures taken to contain it (Heidari et al. 2020; WHO, 2020; UN Women, 2020; Bischof et al., 2020; Wenham et al., 2020).

At the global level, there is a growing political readiness to mainstream gender-based analysis in health research, policy and practice. The World Health Organization, the authority on public health, has a strategy for integrating gender analysis and actions into the work of the WHO that dates back to 2009, adopted as resolution 60.25 at the 60th World Health Assembly (WHA). The WHA urged "Member States to formulate national strategies for addressing gender issues in health policies, programs, research, and planning processes. It also urged the Member States to ensure that a gender-equality perspective is incorporated in all levels of health-care delivery and services. In addition, the resolution requested the Director-General to ensure the full implementation of the strategy" (WHO, 2008b.

p. 2). WHO's Polio Eradication Programme has its own dedicated Gender Equality Strategy (2019–2023), in which it reiterates that it is by "identifying and addressing gender-related barriers to immunization, communication and disease surveillance and to advancing gender equality" that a polio-free world could be realized (WHO, 2019).

Other international organizations such as GAVI, STOP TB Alliance and Global Fund to Fights AIDS, TB and Malaria as well as international and regional non-governmental and private organizations have, to a varied extent, expressed a commitment to mainstream gender in health research, policies and programmes.

Most organizations continue to struggle with the operationalization of their gender policies. One of the key points consistently highlighted in every gender policy is the importance of available evidence and data. The need to prioritize the collection of sex-disaggregated data by national governments, and gender analysis, particularly during the current COVID-19 pandemic, is a consistent pledge by organizations, but one that remains challenging to address (WHO, 2020; GENDRO, 2020). Systematic collection and reporting of data disaggregated by sex and other critical dimensions such as age continues to be "the source of differing and contradictory viewpoints" in many organizations (GAVI 2012).

Mainstreaming gender means that gender is everyone's business. Nevertheless, the responsibility of implementing gender policies at organizational or country level and provision of technical support and capacity building often fall on the shoulders of a gender task force or unit with dedicated expertise. While the approach is critical for strengthening capacity and accountability, it is not gender mainstreaming. In many cases such an approach could even be counterproductive as the gender experts or units tend to be under-resourced, under-funded and often marginalized and disempowered within the organization/institutions, making mainstreaming gender a rather daunting undertaking.

Conclusion

It is no longer possible to dispute the relevance of sex and gender – beyond the binary – in public health research, policy and practice. There is also a high-level political recognition that achieving sustainable development goals, including its ambitious target of universal health coverage, requires gender responsiveness.

During the past decade, we have witnessed a growing number of initiatives that challenge the current health research ecosystem by exposing the risks of gender-blind research not only on women, transgender and gender-non-conforming people who are often overlooked in research, but also on men. Strategic measures have been introduced at different heath research gatekeeping locations and junctures to motivate researchers to incorporate sex and gender and consider their intersection with other social determinants of inequality, as a matter of routine. Several research funding agencies, academic journals, academic institutions and public health organizations actively advocate for sex and gender-based analysis to be an integral part of public health. These efforts are catalysts of change and reasons to be optimistic.

The ongoing COVID-19 pandemic reminds us once again how gender penetrates every aspect of our lives and shapes our physical, mental and social health, and simply cannot be unseen. The aspiration of health for all and the highest attainable standard of health can only be realized through inclusive research with sex and gender in mind, most definitively, if we mean to leave no one behind.

Additional Resources

Instructions for Authors MDPI https://www.mdpi.com/journal/publications/instructions Accessed 20 May 2021.

Springer Editorial Policies: Sex and Gender in Research (SAGER Guidelines) https://www.springer.com/gp/editorial-policies/sex-and-gender-in-research-sager-guidelines Accessed 20 May 2021.

Miles J. (2020). The importance of sex and gender reporting: In support of the SAGER guidelines. https://www.elsevier.com/connect/editors-update/the-importance-of-sex-and-gender-reporting.

References

Adams, N., Pearce, R., Veale, J., Radix, A., Castro, D., & Sarkar, A. (2017). Guidance and ethical considerations for undertaking transgender health research and institutional review boards passing on judicially this research. *Transgender Health, 2*(1), 165–175.

Alzahrani, T., Nguyen, T., Ryan, A., Dwairy, A., McCaffrey, J., & Yunus, R. (2019). Cardiovascular disease risk factors and myocardial infarction in the transgender population. *Cardiovasc Qual Outcomes, 12*(4), 1–7.

Avery, E., & Clark, J. (2016). Sex-related reporting in randomised controlled trials in medical journals. *Lancet, 388*(10062), 2839–2840.

Baptiste-Roberts, K., Oranuba, E., Werts, N., & Edwards, L. V. (2017). Addressing health care disparities among sexual minorities. *Obstetrics and Gynecology Clinics of North America, 44*(1), 71–80.

Bischof, E., Oertelt-Prigione, S., Morgan, R., & Klein, S. (2020). Towards precision medicine: Inclusion of sex and gender aspects in covid-19 clinical studies—Acting now before it is too late—A joint call for action. *International Journal of Environmental Research and Public Health, 17*(10), 3715.

Canadian Institutes of Health Research. (2016). *The ethical imperative of sex and gender considerations in health research.* Available from: https://cihr-irsc.gc.ca/e/49932.html

CIHR Institute of Gender and Health. (2018). *Science is better with sex and gender.* Available from: https://cihr-irsc.gc.ca/e/51310.html

Clayton, J. A., & Collins, F. S. (2014). NIH to balance sex in cell and animal studies. *Nature, 509*(7500), 282–283.

Colpitts, E., & Gahagan, J. (2016). The utility of resilience as a conceptual framework for understanding and measuring LGBTQ health. *International Journal for Equity in Health, 15*, 60.

Committee on Ethical and Legal Issues Relating to the Inclusion of Women in Clinical Studies. (1994). Women and health research: Ethical and legal issues of including women in clinical studies. In A. C. Mastroianni, R. Ruth Faden, & D. F. Federman (Eds.), *Medicine* (Vol. 1).

Committee on the Ethical and Legal Issues Relating to the Inclusion of Women in Clinical Studies Division of Health Sciences Policy Institute of Medicine National.

Curno, M. J., Rossi, S., Hodges-Mameletzis, I., Johnston, R., Price, M. A., & Heidari, S. (2016). A systematic review of the inclusion (or exclusion) of women in HIV research: From clinical studies of antiretrovirals and vaccines to cure strategies. *Journal of Acquired Immune Deficiency Syndromes, 71*(2), 181–188.

Davis, S. L. M. (2017). The uncounted: Politics of data and visibility in global health. *International Journal of Human Rights, 21*(8), 1144–1163.

Directorate-General for Research and Innovation. (2019). She figures 2018. Available from: http://dx.publications.europa.eu/10.2777/936.

EIGE (2015). *Gender equality in academia and research* GEAR tool, EIGE, Lithuania.

European Commission. (2009). *Toolkit: Gender in EU-funded research*. Available from: http://europa.eu

European Commission. (2015). *For a better integration of the gender dimension in Horizon 2020 Work Programme 2016–2017*. Available from: https://ec.europa.eu/transparency/regexpert/index.cfm?do=groupDetail.groupDetailDoc&id=18892&no=1

European Commission. (2020). *Horizon 2020 online manual*. Available from: https://ec.europa.eu/research/participants/docs/h2020-funding-guide/cross-cutting-issues/gender_en.htm

Foulkes, M. A. (2011). After inclusion, information and inference: Reporting on clinical trials results after 15 years of monitoring inclusion of women. *Journal of Women's Health, 20*(6), 829–836.

Gahagan, J., & Colpitts, E. (2017). Understanding and measuring lgbtq pathways to health: A scoping review of strengths-based health promotion approaches in LGBTQ health research. *Journal of Homosexuality, 64*(1), 95–121.

Gahagan, J., Gray, K., & Whynacht, A. (2015). Sex and gender matter in health research: Addressing health inequities in health research reporting. *International Journal for Equity in Health, 14*(1), 12–15.

GAVI. (2012). https://www.gavi.org/our-impact/evaluation-studies/gender-policy-evaluation.

GENDRO. (2020). A call for urgent action: A renewed commitment to gender responsive research for health equity and human rights in the context of COVID-19.

George, A. S., Amin, A., García-Moreno, C., & Sen, G. (2019). Gender equality and health: Laying the foundations for change. *Lancet, 393*(10189), 2369–2371.

Gonzales, G., Przedworski, J., & Henning-Smith, C. (2016). Comparison of health and health risk factors between lesbian, gay, and bisexual adults and heterosexual adults in the United States: Results from the national health interview survey. *JAMA Internal Medicine, 176*(9), 1344–1351.

Government of Canada. (2009). Health Portfolio sex and gender-based analysis policy. *Public Health*. Available from: http://www.hc-sc.gc.ca/hl-vs/pubs/women-femmes/sgba-policy-politique-ags-eng.php

Government of Canada Minister of Health. (2000). *Health Canada's gender-based analysis policy*.

Hankivsky, O. (2012). Women's health, men's health, and gender and health: Implications of intersectionality. *Social Science & Medicine, 74*(11), 1712–1720.

Hankivsky, O., Springer, K. W., & Hunting, G. (2018). Beyond sex and gender difference in funding and reporting of health research. *Research Integrity and Peer Review, 3*(1), 6.

Heidari, S., & Bachelet, V. C. (2018). Sex and gender analysis for better science and health equity. *Lancet, 392*(10157), 1500.

Heidari, S., & Doyle, H. (2020). An invitation to a feminist approach to global health data. *Health and Human Rights Journal, 22*(2), 75–78.

Heidari S, Ahumada C, Kurbanova Z, et al. Towards the real-time inclusion of sex- and age-disaggregated data in pandemic responses. BMJ Global Health 2020;5:e003848. https://doi.org/10.1136/bmjgh-2020-003848.

Heidari, S., Eckert, M. J., Kippax, S., Karim, Q., Sow, P., & Wainberg, M. A. (2011). Time for gender mainstreaming in editorial policies. *Journal of the International AIDS Society, 14*(1), 11.

Heidari, S., Abdool Karim, Q., Auerbach, J. D., Buitendijk, S. E., Cahn, P., & Curno, M. J. (2012). Gender-sensitive reporting in medical research. *Journal of the International AIDS Society, 15*(1), 11.

Heidari, S., Babor, T. F., De Castro, P., Tort, S., & Curno, M. (2016). Sex and gender equity in research: Rationale for the SAGER guidelines and recommended use. *Research Integrity & Peer Review, 1*(1), 319–320.

Helsinki Group on Gender in Research and Innovation Position. (2017). *Position paper on H2020 interim evaluation and preparation of FP9*. Available from: https://s3-eu-west-1.amazonaws.com/data.epws.org/EPWS+NEWSPAGE/2017/HG+position+paper_H2020+interim+evaluation_adopted.pdf

Holdcroft, A. (2007). Gender bias in research: How does it affect evidence based medicine? *Journal of the Royal Society of Medicine, 100*(1), 2–3.

Horton, R. (2019). Offline: Gender and global health—An inexcusable global failure. *Lancet, 393*(10171), 511.

Human Rights Watch. (2018). *US: LGBT people face healthcare barriers | Human Rights Watch*. Available from: https://www.hrw.org/news/2018/07/23/us-lgbt-people-face-healthcare-barriers. Accessed 20 August 2020

Institute of Medicine (US) Committee on Ethical and Legal Issues Relating to the Inclusion of Women in Clinical Studies. Women and Health Research: Ethical and Legal Issues of Including Women in Clinical Studies: Volume I. Mastroianni AC, Faden R, Federman D, editors. Washington (DC): National Academies Press (US); 1994. PMID: 25144026. https://doi.org/10.17226/2304

Johnson, J., Sharman, Z., Vissandjée, B., & Stewart, D. E. (2014). Does a change in health research funding policy related to the integration of sex and gender have an impact? *PLoS One, 9*(6), e99900. Available from: https://dx.plos.org/10.1371/journal.pone.0099900

Kim, A. M., Tingen, C. M., & Woodruff, T. K. (2010). Sex bias in trials and treatment must end. *Nature, 465*(7299), 688–689.

The Lancet. (2008). The Bamako call to action: research for health. *Lancet, 372*(9653):1855.

Lancet. (2018). Gender and health are also about boys and men. *Lancet, 392*(10143), 188.

Lawrence, K., & Rieder, A. (2007). Methodologic and ethical ramifications of sex and gender differences in public health research. *Gender Medicine, 4*(SUPPL. 2), S96.

Lyerly, A. D., Little, M. O., & Faden, R. (2008). The second wave: Toward responsible inclusion of pregnant women in research. *International Journal of Feminist Approaches to Bioethics, 1*(2), 5–22.

Mastroianni, A. C., Faden, R., & Federman, D. (1994). Women and health research: A report from the Institute of Medicine. *Kennedy Institute of Research Ethics Journal, 4*(1), 55–62.

Matthen, P., Lyons, T., Taylor, M., Jennex, J., Anderson, S., & Jollimore, J. (2018). "I walked into the industry for survival and came out of a closet": How gender and sexual identities shape sex work experiences among men, two Spirit, and trans people in Vancouver. *Men and Masculinities, 21*(4), 479–500.

Mayer, K. H., Bradford, J. B., Makadon, H. J., Stall, R., Goldhammer, H., & Landers, S. (2008). Sexual and gender minority health: What we know and what needs to be done. *American Journal of Public Health, 98*(6), 989–995.

Merton, R. K. (1973). *The sociology of science: Theoretical and empirical investigations*. Storer: The University of Chicago Press.

Mexico Statement on Health Research. (2004). *Knowledge for better health : Strengthening health systems*. From The Ministerial Summit On Health Research.

Ministerial Summit on Health Research. (2004). https://apps.who.int/gb/archive/pdf_files/EB115/B115_30-en.pdf.

Morselli, E., Frank, A. P., Santos, R. S., Fátima, L. A., Palmer, B. F., & Clegg, D. J. (2016). Sex and gender: Critical variables in pre-clinical and clinical medical research. *Cell Metabolism, 24*(2), 203–209.

National Institutes of Health. (1993). *National Institutes of Health Revitalization Act of 1993*. Available from: http://orwh.od.nih.gov/about/pdf/NIH-Revitalization-Act-1993.pdf

National Institutes of Health. (2018). *Task force on research specific to pregnant women and lactating women*. Available from: https://www.nichd.nih.gov/about/advisory/PRGLAC

National Research Act. (1974). https://www.govinfo.gov/content/pkg/STATUTE-88/pdf/STATUTE-88-Pg342.pdf#page=5.

Nature. (2010). Putting gender on the agenda. *Nature, 465*(7299), 665–665. Available from: http://www.nature.com/articles/465665a

Palmer-Ross A, Ovseiko PV, Heidari S Inadequate reporting of COVID-19 clinical studies: a renewed rationale for the Sex and Gender Equity in Research (SAGER) guidelines BMJ Global Health 2021;6:e004997. http://dx.doi.org/10.1136/bmjgh-2021-004997.

Pinn VW. (2003). Sex and gender factors in medical studies: implications for health and clinical practice. *JAMA, 289*(4):397–400.

Purnell, B., Roberts, L., & Smith, O. (2005). Vive la différence. *Science, 308*(June), 1569.

Ramasubbu, H., Gurm, D., & Litaker, M. (2001). Gender bias in clinical trials: Do double standards still apply? *Journal of Womens Health & Gender Based Medicine, 10*(8), 757–764.

Rásky, É., Waxenegger, A., Groth, S., Stolz, E., Schenouda, M., & Berzlanovich, A. (2017). Sex and gender matters. *Wiener Klinische Wochenschrift, 129*(21–22), 781–785.

Reisner, S. L., Poteat, T., Keatley, J., Cabral, M., Mothopeng, T., & Dunham, E. (2016). Global health burden and needs of transgender populations: A review. *Lancet, 388*(10042), 412–436.

Rio Political Declaration on Social Determinants of Health. (2011). 14(October), 1–7.

Schiebinger, L. (2003). Women's health and clinical trials. *Journal of Clinical Investigation*, (7), 973–977.

Schiebinger, L., Leopold, S. S., & Miller, V. M. (2016). Editorial policies for sex and gender analysis. *Lancet, 388*(10062), 2841–2842.

Schneider, M.-J. (2012). *Introduction to public health*. Sudbury: Jones and Bartlett Publishers.

Scientific Advisory Board of the UN Secretary-General. (2016). *Science for sustainable development: Policy brief*. Available from: http://unesdoc.unesco.org/images/0024/002461/246104E.pdf

Sen, G., Östlin, P., & George, A. (2007). *Unequal, unfair, ineffective and inefficient ghender inequity in health : Why it exists and how we can change it*. Final Report to the WHO Commission on Social Determinants of Health Women and Gender Equity Knowledge Network Gita Sen and Piroska Östlin Rev. World Health. 1–145.

Sen, G., Reddy, B., Iyer, A., & Heidari, S. (2018a). Addressing disrespect and abuse during childbirth in facilities. *Reproductive Health Matters, 26*(53), 1–5.

Sen, G., Reddy, B., & Iyer, A. (2018b). Beyond measurement: The drivers of disrespect and abuse in obstetric care. *Reproductive Health Matters, 26*(53a), 6–18.

Sherman, L. A., Temple, R., & Merkatz, R. B. (1995). Women in clinical trials: An FDA perspective. *Science, 269*(5225), 793–795.

Taylor, E., & Bryson, M. K. (2016). Cancer's Margins: Trans* and gender nonconforming people's access to knowledge, experiences of cancer health, and decision-making. *LGBT Health, 3*(1), 79–89.

Tulchinsky, T. H., Varavikova, E. A., & Bickford, J. D. (2015). *The new public health* (New Public Heal 3 ed.). Elsevier Academic Press.

UNFPA. (2020, March). *Covid-19: A gender lens. Protecting sexual and reproductive health and rights, and promoting gender equality*. Available from: https://www.unfpa.org/sites/default/files/resource-pdf/COVID-19_A_Gender_Lens_Guidance_Note.pdf

United Nations General Assembly. (2014). https://unstats.un.org/unsd/dnss/gp/fp-new-e.pdf.

United Nations. (2017). *Global indicator framework for the Sustainable Development Goals and targets of the 2030 Agenda for Sustainable Development*. Available from: https://unstats.un.org/sdgs/indicators/GlobalIndicatorFrameworkafterrefinement_Eng.pdf

UN Women. (2020). *Policy Brief: The impact of COVID-19 on women*. Available from: file:///C:/Users/camiv/Downloads/Policy-brief-the-impact-of-covid-19-on-women-en (1).pdf.

Weber, A. M., Cislaghi, B., Meausoone, V., Abdalla, S., Mejía-Guevara, I., & Loftus, P. (2019). Gender norms and health: Insights from global survey data. *Lancet, 393*(10189), 2455–2468.

Welch, V., Doull, M., Yoganathan, M., Jull, J., Boscoe, M., & Coen, S. E. (2017). Reporting of sex and gender in randomized controlled trials in Canada: A cross-sectional methods study. *Research Integrity and Peer Review, 2*(1), 15.

Wenham, C., Smith, J., & Morgan, R. (2020). COVID-19: The gendered impacts of the outbreak. *Lancet, 395*(10227), 846–848.

Wenneras, C., & Wold, A. (1997). Nepotism and sexism in peer-review. *Nature, 387,* 341.

Winter, S., Diamond, M., Green, J., Karasic, D., Reed, T., & Whittle, S. (2016). Transgender people: Health at the margins of society. *Lancet, 388*(10042), 390–400.

Witter, S., Govender, V., Ravindran, T. S., & Yates, R. (2017). Minding the gaps: Health financing, universal health coverage and gender. *Health Policy and Plannning, 32*(Suppl_5), v4–12.

Wizemann, T. M. (2012). *Sex-specific reporting of scientific research.* The National Academies Press.

World Health Organization. (2005). *World Health Assembly Resolution 58.34* Ministerial Summit on Health Research. Available from: https://apps.who.int/iris/bitstream/handle/10665/20384/WHA58_34-en.pdf?sequence=1

World Health Organization. (2008a). *Strategy for integrating gender analysis and action into the work of the WHO.*

World Health Organization. (2008b, Nov 17–19). *The Bamako call to action on research for health. Strengthening research for health, development, and equity.* Global research for Health. From the global Ministerial Forum on Research for Health, Bamako, Mali.

World Health Organization. (2019). *Breaking barriers: Towards more gender-responsive and equitable health systems.*

World Health Organization. (2020). *Gender and COVID-19: Advocacy brief.* Available from: https://apps.who.int/iris/handle/10665/332080

World Health Organization and Office of the United Nations High Commissioner for Human Rights. (2008).*The right to health.* Available from: https://www.who.int/gender-equity-rights/knowledge/right-to-health-factsheet31.pdf?ua=1

Chapter 3
Sex- and Gender-Based Analyses and Advancing Population Health

Natisha Dukhi, Priscilla Reddy, and Nompumelelo Zungu

The State of Population Health Globally and Context for Why SGBA Is Critical for Advancing Population Health

Population health is defined as an interdisciplinary approach that has an increased focus on health outcomes as well as the roles and interactions of the health determinants, which influence the health of populations over the life course (Kindig & Stoddart, 2003). Traditionally, healthcare delivery has focused on the care and needs of the individual. For the advancement of health, both individual and public health must be integrated. Population health evolved, with a focus on the measurement of the determinants and optimization of the health of populations (Gourevitch, 2014; Ruiz & Verbrugge, 1997). The population health approach encompasses the study of interrelated conditions and factors (i.e. physical, social, and economic factors) influencing the health of a population over time. It also focuses on the identification of differences in occurrence patterns and uses knowledge generated for the development and implementation of interventions and policies for the improvement of health and well-being in populations (Dunn & Hayes, 1999). The approach informs how interventions can be designed, implemented, monitored, and evaluated, as well as who it specifically targets. This in turn allows for the health status of the population to be improved and may also result in a decline of health inequities among these populations (Federal Advisory Committee on Population Health, 1994; Public Health Agency of Canada, 2001). The approach accounts for sex and gender in population health and will assist

N. Dukhi (✉) · P. Reddy
Human and Social Capabilities, Human Sciences Research Council, Pretoria, South Africa
e-mail: ndukhi@hsrc.ac.za

N. Zungu
Human and Social Capabilities, Human Sciences Research Council, Pretoria, South Africa

Department of Psychology, University of Pretoria, Pretoria, South Africa

© Springer Nature Switzerland AG 2021
J. Gahagan, M. K. Bryson (eds.), *Sex- and Gender-Based Analysis in Public Health*, https://doi.org/10.1007/978-3-030-71929-6_3

researchers and policymakers to develop practices that will also assist in addressing health disparities (Clow et al., 2009; Johnson et al., 2007).

There is increasing health research promoting sex- and gender-based analyses (SGBA), as well as how sex and gender both influence health behaviours and health outcomes (Krieger, 2003; Lawrence & Rieder, 2007; Vlassoff & Moreno, 2002). Despite sex and gender receiving increased attention, the effective application of both these concepts is often conflated and used interchangeably or altogether absent in health research (Johnson et al., 2009; Krieger, 2003). As a result, the unique and intersecting contributions of sex and gender in health outcomes are often insufficiently addressed in the data analyses and dissemination, leading to missed opportunities to develop and implement appropriate population health interventions and policies (Krieger, 2003). The inclusion of sex and gender in health research not only contributes to better science, but it also ensures that healthcare systems address challenges of social justice, ethics, and equity (Aulakh & Anand, 2007; Gesensway, 2001; Greaves et al., 1999).

Sex is a biological construct that is multidimensional and refers to the biological characteristics such as the anatomy (body shape and size) and the physiology (organ functioning or hormonal activity) that is often used to distinguish cisgender males from cisgender females (Health Canada, 2003; Public Health Agency of Canada, 2012). It is important to note that sex is often referred to in binary terms such as male and female or man and woman, but the attributes of sex, which include chromosomal differences and hormone level variations, are often described to exist on a continuum (Canadian Institutes of Health Research, 2012; Johnson et al., 2009). Gender, on the other hand, is often referred to as a social and multidimensional construct, manifesting at many levels. It is culturally based and constructed of relationships and roles, behaviours, attitudes, influence, and values that society attributes to the male and female sexes (Health Canada, 2000). The concept of gender is also expressed in gender identity. It informs how we define ourselves in the gender identity spectrum and related societal interactions (Teich, 2012). Gender identity is often constructed as a binary and tends to account for cisgender individuals, leaving out other gender identities such as transgender and gender diverse individuals who do not follow the typical feminine nor masculine conventions (Rider et al., 2018).

SGBA is based on the understanding that both sex and gender affect our lives and health at the level of the individual and at the population health level. Importantly, it challenges the tendency to apply "one size fits all" and explores differences and similarities by sex and gender and accounts for variations (Clow et al., 2009). In health research specifically, different sexes and genders may have different risk profiles, responses, and uptake of intervention-based various sociodemographic and locality-type variables. Health conditions and/or access to health services need to also factor context and culture in explaining poor health outcomes. SGBA urges researchers, policymakers, and population health programme implementers to analyse the health inequities that arise from gender relations, how these intersect with other determinants, and how these can influence how individuals respond to the health system (Clow et al., 2009; Day et al., 2016).

The Core Concepts of Sex- and Gender-Based Analysis Within the Context of Broader Determinants of Health

The four core concepts of SGBA include sex, gender, diversity, and equity (Clow et al., 2009). These core concepts together create a framework for examining diversity in the experience of both health and illness, as well as evaluating the extent to which the health system responds effectively, efficiently, fairly, and equally (Johnson et al., 2009). It accounts for observable sociodemographic differences and other evident differences such as spiritual or religious persuasion and sexual orientation. Within the SGBA context, it is understood that individuals develop gender identity and enact gender and may experience health problems that are gender-related in the same way (Clow et al., 2009). By exploring diversity using SGBA, one can identify and offer potential solutions for inequities in health.

In relation to the core concept of equity in SGBA, health inequities are defined as a contrast in health outcomes which are avoidable, unfair, and/or changeable (Pan American Health Organization, 1999). Health inequities are experienced when an individual or population suffers a greater burden of illness or the severity of the illness is increased due to social injustice (Labonte et al., 2005; Raphael, 2004). Social hierarchies and related socioeconomic and demographic factors affect who are at risk of illness and whose long-term economic, personal, and social outlook will be most affected by ill health. It is such issues that will define the boundaries of the analyses, discussions, and conclusions drawn (Day et al., 2016; Public Health Agency of Canada, 2012).

Advantages and Challenges of Incorporating Sex- and Gender-Based Analysis in Population Health Research

Worldwide, research funding bodies are mandating researchers to address sex and gender in their proposals as a requirement to fulfil before awarding funding (Johnson & Beaude, 2013). This shift reflects the importance research has showed differences in physiological and hormonal makeup by sex (Johnson et al., 2009) making it imperative to include sex variables in research. Gender, by definition, dictates the roles and how individuals interact and are treated by others. Sex and gender are critical elements for understanding health behaviours and health outcomes within the population. In different societies, being male or female is generally defined and interpreted differently; thus, susceptibility to environmental risk, occupational risks, access to health care, risk-taking behaviours, and utilization patterns of health care differ as a result (Johnson & Beaude, 2013).

Sex and gender are fundamental mechanisms through which a distinction can be made or conclusions reached regarding diagnoses and treatments offered. For example, due to physiological and social factors cisgender, heterosexual women face across the life course, and they have historically been categorized as more vulnerable to certain diseases such as HIV infection as compared to men (UNAIDS, 2019), with an exception of men who have sex with men (UNAIDS, 2019). Analyses that include sex and gender assist in finding the solutions and development of relevant interventions (Mayer et al., 2008). Specifically, prior to the promotion of SGBA, most clinical trials for HIV medications included male subjects only, and thus opportunities were missed in investigating how women living with HIV would respond to the same medications. It was later discovered that pharmacodynamics and pharmaceutical agents differ between sexes (Heidari et al., 2016). For instance, a study on aspirin that had a majority representation of men led to wrong conclusions that aspirin was effective on men only. The equal effectiveness of aspirin on women was discovered later on and women started to benefit later than men (Johnson et al., 2009). Therefore, SGBA fosters understanding on the variation of impact of drugs between men and women and helps to decode healthcare utilization patterns that affect health outcomes (Nowatzki & Grant, 2010). Doing research that disregards SGBA can lead to skewed representation and pose a challenge to replicate findings in other settings.

Using SGBA can also be problematic by paying more attention to one sex or specific health issues. This can lead to certain diseases being assocaited with a particular sex such as HIV (Bird & Rieker, 1999). Research has revealed men's higher risk for developing heart disease early in life (Khayyam-Nekouei et al., 2013). As a result of gender aggregates, men and women face particular stereotypical responses regarding masculinity-related issues: identities and risk behaviours that may perpetuate unhealthy patriarchal practices that can be damaging to efforts to reverse this notion (Doyal, 2001). Likewise, women may face stigmatization as weaker citizens, disadvantaged by their physiological makeup to be susceptible to disease (Visser et al., 2009). This could reinforce prevalent notions that make women in a continuous cycle of vulnerability (Bowleg, 2012). If the science is not carefully developed or its interpretation accurate, such analysis may validate gendered perspectives of prowess and hegemony or conflict between sexes which makes individual, family-level, and societal cohesion challenging and can promote inequality (Ovseiko et al., 2016). However, including intersectional variables such as sex and gender, among others, in health research "may complicate things" (Hankivsky & Christoffersen, 2008).

Although there is a plethora of evidence on the value that SGBA in health research can offer, there are ambiguities with definitions and methodological approaches. As mentioned previously, gender is often confused with sex (Runnels et al., 2014). The SGBA process should therefore include information and evidence sources such as surveys, statistical analyses, interviews, case studies, consultations, and media coverage in research (Clow et al., 2009). It has been suggested that traditional evidence in the form of quantitative data is preferred by healthcare decision-makers, health researchers, and policymakers alike and this can contribute to understanding sex and gender, as well as other key determinants of health (Gopalakrishnan & Ganeshkumar, 2013).

Despite the growing consensus that SGBA makes for better science, researchers have noted that a simple acknowledgment of gender is limiting and provides no guidance on how changes can be made in different health programmes. Gender sensitivity refers to the ways in which a research project, intervention, or policy is designed in response to gender roles and the relations which mark attitudes and behaviours of participants and how they may influence the outcomes (UNICEF, 2011). To frame the research question in gender-sensitive research, a gender analytical framework can be used, or it can involve the inclusion of thinking through potential gender issues before proceeding with the research. In gender-sensitive research, various factors must be considered. These include research topics and their relevance to problems and needs, consideration of gender training for research staff and those collecting data, the acknowledging of differences between the researchers and participants, and data collectors and/or researchers/participants, whereby these differences can lead to poor health or treatment outcomes. Other factors include incorporation of multiple data collection methods to allow both women and men participants to tell their own stories; to improve the welfare of the participants and not just use data as part of the publication process, allowing the participants to voluntarily participate in the research process; to respect and maintain confidentiality; as well as to not be coercive but rather allowing participants their right to abstain from answering any questions or participating in any component of the project (UNICEF, 2011). New research protocols and survey tools, inclusive of the earlier mentioned factors, are required so that researchers and policymakers are enabled to address with understanding the four core concepts of SGBA. However, such a transition will take time and require effort (Day et al., 2016).

The emergence of innovative methods for health analyses creates an interesting opportunity to look into SGBA theory and practice in population health and show how this can be expanded. One such area that has the potential to shape SGBA is the core concepts within the context of the broader determinants of health (Public Health Agency of Canada, 2012). In some countries, gender is recognized as a determinant of health, but it is not clearly linked to the other health determinants. Both sex and gender interact with the various other determinants of health that influence population health (Day et al., 2016). These determinants of health, of which some have been mentioned before, include social status, income, education, employment, physical environments such as community infrastructure and housing, social environments such as the workplace and community, culture that includes cultural and racial identities, child development, and health service. These determinants can influence behaviours, outcomes, health risks, and/or opportunities during the different stages of life (Gaudet, 2007). While each health determinant contributes to health outcomes, the intersections between these creates various complex contexts in which the choices are made at the level of the indiviudal can affect health outcomes within and across populations (Greaves, 2011).

Population Health Research and SGBA: A Case of Study of the HIV and AIDS Epidemic in South Africa – Lessons from the South African National HIV, Behaviour, and Communication Survey

As noted earlier there has been an international push for gender to be included in the research impact assessment conducted by research funders, institutions, and evaluators in order to inform more equitable health policy and practice (Day et al., 2016; Ovseiko et al., 2016). The challenges of including SGBA are more prominent in the HIV and AIDS research, policymaking, and implementation. South Africa has continued to have the highest number of people living with HIV and AIDS in the world, and AIDS has remained one of the leading courses of death, representing a significant burden to the health system. The remainder of this chapter focuses on HIV and AIDS as a unique case study illustrating the importance of including SGBA in population health research.

South Africa has tracked the progression of the HIV epidemic using the household survey, among other tools, since 2002 (Shisana & Simbayi, 2002). The Fifth South African National Prevalence, Incidence, Behaviour and Communication Survey (SABSSM V) was conducted by a consortium led by the Human Sciences Research Council (HSRC) between 2016 and 2017. SABSSM is recognized globally for its contribution to the monitoring and surveillance of the HIV epidemic in the country (Simbayi et al., 2019). We will use data from this survey to illustrate the nexus between SGBA, population health research, and policy development (see Shisana et al., 2005, 2009, 2014; Shisana & Simbayi, 2002; Simbayi et al., 2019). We will also illustrate how this survey has successfully provided data that is disaggregated by sex, to a limited extent sexual orientation, and how these data have informed the response. We will also highlight that although the role of SGBA in the formulation of policies that are sensitive to sex and gender is recognized, this remains a challenge not only in South Africa but globally. The planned 2021 SABSSM VI survey, aimed at bridging the SGBA gap, will include gender-specific questions that will allow for a more nuanced analysis of HIV data going forward.

The prevalence of HIV has continued to increase over time (12.2% in 2012) and was estimated to be 14.0%, which translated into an estimated 7.9 million people living with HIV in 2017 (Simbayi et al., 2019). Black Africans continue to carry the highest burden of HIV, with Black African cisgender, heterosexual women aging 20–34 having the highest HIV prevalence and incidence per year (Shisana et al., 2014; Simbayi et al., 2019). Although race is not the focus of SGBA, the intersection between race and sex cannot be ignored as it is a key determinant of HIV acquisition and studying it is critical for understanding social determinants related to health equity and health disparity challenges. It has been suggested that equity in particular is the ultimate driver of sex- and gender-based analysis. Clow et al. (2009) have argued that "health inequities – like other forms of inequity – are often rooted in differences of power and privilege distributed along the fault lines of sex, gender and diversity" (p.158). Indeed experience has shown that research, policies, and programmes that do not account for these key variables will fail to redress health inequities and may, in fact, have the unintended consequence of deepening the existing disparities or even creating new ones (Clow et al., 2009). This will be demonstrated later in this chapter with regard to the use of data for targeting adolescent girls and young women and the impact of this on the HIV incidence among men (Simbayi et al., 2019).

HIV Prevalence and Incidence: The Tale of Sex Differences

Sex-based analysis conducted routinely as part SABSSM survey has provided valuable strategic information that has improved not only our understanding of the epidemiology of HIV but has also informed the response to fighting HIV and AIDS in South Africa. The five surveys (Shisana et al., 2005, 2009, 2014; Shisana & Simbayi, 2002; Simbayi et al., 2019) demonstrated the impact of HIV among cisgender, heterosexual females and to a limited extent the role of gender in the continued spread of HIV in the country. Data has demonstrated the increase in risk for Black South African cisgender heterosexual women, particularly younger women (Dellar et al., 2015; Kenyon et al., 2016; Shisana et al., 2015). Adolescent heterosexual cisgender girls and young women (AGYW) aged 15–24 years remain at high risk for HIV infection, with a prevalence estimated to be eight times that of their heterosexual male counterparts (Dellar et al., 2015; Shisana et al., 2015). Although the epidemic in South Africa is generalized, certain populations are classified as vulnerable or high-risk groups (Shisana et al., 2014, 2015) where HIV prevalence among these groups is higher than that found in the general population. These populations include heterosexual cisgender Black African women aging 20–35, cohabiting heterosexual couples; Black heterosexual cisgender African men aging 25–49; persons with disabilities aged 15 and older; high-risk alcohol drinkers aged 15 and older; and recreational drug users (for prevalence figures in these groups, see Shisana et al., 2014, 2015; Simbayi et al., 2019).

In the 2017 SABSSM V survey, HIV prevalence peaked at 39.4% in the 35–39-year age group among heterosexual, cisgender women. Whereas among heterosexual cisgender men, it peaked at 24.8% in the 45–49-year age group. In all the adult age categories, cisgender females carried a disproportionately higher burden of HIV compared to males. Statistically significant differences were observed by sex from the 20–24-year age group through to the 40–44-year age group. Notably, cisgender women in these age groups had a prevalence that was higher than the prevalence observed nationally. As an example, heterosexual cisgender women aging 20–24 years had an HIV prevalence of 15.6% compared to 4.8% among men ($p < 0.001$) (Simbayi et al., 2019).

The differences by sex emerged even among heterosexual couples when serodiscordancy was investigated in a national HIV prevalence survey (Simbayi et al., 2019). These differences remain even though data on sexual risky behaviour suggests that men are more likely to engage in risky sexual behaviour compared to women (Seth et al., 2012). Of the 1693 heterosexual cisgender couples who provided blood specimens in the 2017 HIV household survey, 11.3% were sero-discordant. Discordancy involving a female HIV-positive and a male HIV-negative partner was more than double at 7.9%. Discordancy where the male partner was HIV-positive and the female was HIV-negative was 3.4%. The data presented earlier show how heterosexual cisgender women are disproportionately affected by HIV and AIDS and that this impact starts very early and peaks around the reproductive age (Simbayi et al., 2019).

Although new infections among heterosexual cisgender adults had declined by 54% from 1999 to 2017, HIV incidence had remained high, with an estimated 253,081 new HIV infections reported in 2017 (incidence based on modelling – Johnson et al., 2017). Evidence demonstrates that rates of new infections, although on the decline, remain high in South Africa. The overall HIV incidence for 2017 for people ages 2 and older was 0.48% (95% CI: 0.42–0.54), and this translated to an estimated 231,100 new infections. A higher proportion of infections occurred among females compared to males. Similar to the 2012 survey (Shisana et al., 2014), heterosexual youth ages 15–24 years had the highest incidence, at an estimated 88,400 new infections in 2017. Geographically, HIV incidence was higher in urban areas (0.58%) than that in rural areas (0.23%). The data also showed early evidence of targeting with declines in incidence more profound in females compared to males. When the 2012 results were recalculated using the 2017 incidence test parameters, the overall HIV incidence has significantly dropped by 44% in the age 2 and older. The largest decline (56%) in incidence was among females. Among males in the same age group, the incidence declined by 18% only, suggesting a need to ensure that cisgender males are not left behind in the country's HIV prevention response (Simbayi et al., 2019).

When data for individuals 15–24 years was examined, the overall HIV incidence among youth declined by 17%. The decline in incidence was again observed among heterosexual cisgender females (26%), and of concern the data showed that among heterosexual cisgender males, the incidence had increased by 11% pointing to the complexity in controlling the epidemic and possible unintended consequences of using data to target heterosexual cisgender adolescent girls and young women aged 15–24 years (AGYW) with interventions, while leaving heterosexual cisgender boys and young men in the same group largely unattended by prevention interventions. An analysis of the reproductive age group 15–49 years found that the overall HIV incidence in the reproductive age group has dropped significantly by 42%. However, the biggest decline (49%) in incidence was among females. Among males the incidence declined by 28%. What incidence data show is that the overall profile of HIV incidence had remained the same, with higher rates among youth, especially young females, and among single individuals and people living in urban areas (Simbayi et al., 2019).

Sex Difference in Behavioural Determinants of HIV

Certain behaviours are considered key drivers of the HIV epidemic in South Africa. Evidence has shown that the risk of HIV infection is associated with certain socio-behavioural and structural factors. These include multiple sexual partners (MSPs), age-disparate sexual relations (Evans et al., 2016, 2017; Shisana et al., 2014), inconsistent condom use, high mobility, migration, exposure to sexual violence, and alcohol use (Madiba & Ngwenya, 2017; McGrath et al.; Pitpitan et al., 2016).

Age at sexual debut is an important determinant of HIV infection. Initiating sex before the age of 15 years is associated with risks to sexual and reproductive health outcomes for both sexes (Richter et al., 2015). South African studies have shown that three times more males than females reported having sex for the first time before the age of 15 (Martinez & Abma, 2015; Shisana et al., 2014). SABBSM V found high rates of early sexual debut among males when compared to females in 2012 and 2017, respectively (Shisana et al., 2015; Simbayi et al., 2019). Fewer than 10% of 15–24-year-olds stated that they had had early sexual debuts. Across the five SABSSM survey rounds, early sexual debut was more common among males than females (Shisana & Simbayi, 2002, Shisana et al., 2005, Shisana et al., 2009, 2014; Simbayi et al., 2019).

Age-disparate relationships have emerged as a key determinant of HIV especially among young women and often reflect the power dynamics that are related to one's gender. Previous surveys have shown that age-disparate sexual relationships, defined as a partner having an age gap of 5 years or more, are associated with increased risk for HIV infection among AGYW (De Oliveira et al., 2016; Evans et al., 2016, 2017; Maughan-Brown et al., 2016). In the SABSSM V study, age-disparate relationships were consistently common among females than males (35.8% females and males 1.5%). Furthermore, fewer males had age-disparate relationships compared to females in the 2012 survey. An upward trend was observed among females since 2005 (18.5%), which means that more women are currently engaged in relationships with older partners (35.8% in 2012) (Shisana et al., 2009, 2014; Simbayi et al., 2019).

Multiple sexual partners (MSP) have been shown to increase the spread of HIV especially during the acute and early infection phases (Pines et al., 2016; UNAIDS, 2015). The SABSSM surveys show that males are more likely than females to report having MSPs among all age groups ages 15 and older (Shisana et al., 2009, 2014; Simbayi et al., 2019). Although these relationships remain prevalent among males ages 15–24 years, a decline was noted in self-reported MSPs among males from 37.5% in 2012 to 25.5% in 2017 (Simbayi et al., 2019). Among females, there has been an increasing trend since 2008 in the 15–49-year age range, being prominent in the age group 15–24 years (8.2–9.0%).

Consistent condom use remains the key for HIV prevention; however, this is among the areas where power comes into play between men and women, with women reporting refusal of men or their fear of suggesting barriers to condom use (Campbell et al., 2016). In spite of the reported barriers to condom use, self-reported condom use at the last sexual activity has been generally higher among males than females across all age groups in South Africa. In the age group 15–24 years for males, it was 67.5%, and for females, it was 49.8%; among the age group 25–49 years, it was 40.2% for males and 36.1% for females, and among ages 50 and older, it was 15.5% for males and 13.8% for females.

Medical male circumcision is the main intervention that is male focused globally. In South Africa there has been a steady increase in the number of men who are circumcised since it was promoted for reducing the risk of HIV infection among men. Since 2002, the proportion of circumcised males ages 15 and older has increased from 38.2% in 2002 to 61.6% in 2017. By 2017, the number of adult males reporting that they had been medically circumcised rose steadily from 1,582,000 in 2002 to 2,269,000 in 2008, 3,301,000 in 2012, and 4,330,000 in 2017. Overall, 13.6% of male children younger than 15 years of age had been circumcised, with the majority of them (89.9%) having had it performed in medical settings (Simbayi et al., 2019).

Intimate partner violence (IPV) is often imbedded in cultural and power relations and is one of the drivers of HIV infection especially among women.[1] For both sexes, the most commonly reported acts of intimate partner violence (IPV) included being pushed, being shaken, having an object thrown at them (12.9%), and being slapped (12.9%). As has been observed in a previous study (Shisana et al., 2014), a higher proportion of females reported experiencing IPV when compared to males. The exception was violence where there was a threat of the use of a weapon or an actual weapon was used, which is a feature that has been observed in other gender-based studies (Abrahams et al., 2010). Physical violence was experienced frequently by 1.3% of people, with females reporting slightly higher proportions (1.6%) than males (1.1%). Males and females reported IPV showed a higher prevalence of HIV-positive status than people who did not report IPV. For males, the difference in HIV status was significant (28.6% vs 14.1%; $p = 0.001$) (Simbayi et al., 2019).

Where Are the Cisgender Men in the HIV and AIDS Interventions? Sex-Based Disparities in Key HIV and AIDS Indicators

There is a growing body of knowledge in the area of masculinities that explains how gender impacts men's health (Connell, 1987, 1995; Courtenay, 2000; Mfecane, 2018). Men's health as a field of study emerged in the 1980s from a need to generate evidence on how gender-based assumptions about, for example, health-seeking behaviours among men create unique understandings of the pathways to health care as well as how they are treated (Clow et al., 2009). Similar to women's health research, men's health research has been motivated by an absence of gender-based

---

[1] The IPV scale measured both the current and past experience and perpetration of violence. Men and women who were ever in an intimate relationship responded to questions about their "partner."

analysis and the presumption that "what it means to be a man … has no bearing on how men work, drink, drive, fight, or take risks" (Courtenay, 2000, p. 1387). Indeed, studies that investigate health risks that are more common to men than women often exclude gender as a central factor (Clow et al., 2009).

It is important to note that data show that access to HIV interventions differs along lines of sex and gender in that heterosexual cisgender males are less likely to be reached by such HIV and AIDS interventions compared to their female counterparts, particularly females within reproductive age (UNAIDS, 2016). Further, while the UNAIDS 90–90–90 strategy identifies HIV testing as the key entry point for initiating those who test positive to HIV on antiretroviral treatment (ART) and for achieving viral load (VL) suppression and thereby reducing the onward transmission of the virus (UNAIDS, 2014), an analysis of HIV testing and treatment data suggests serious health disparities with regard to access and reach by sex. When exposure to ART was investigated, the data showed that the number of people living with HIV on ART had increased, with 62.3% receiving ART, which translated into an estimated 4.4 million people receiving ART in South Africa in 2017. However, an analysis by sex shows that the success of ART is not equitable. Proportionately more females (65.5%) were on ART compared to males (56.3%); this is a long-standing gendered disparity. It should be noted that the disparities in the uptake of ART are mostly related to women within reproductive age being more regularly screened as part of the global focus on reducing HIV incidence among AGYW and also as part of reducing mother to child transmission to zero (MTCT). However, among males there is no comparable sexual reproductive men's health intervention targeting heterosexual males (UNAIDS, 2016), and HIV interventions largely depend on influencing men's decision-making to influence health-seeking behaviour, something that has been difficult to achieve.

Although men may not be as well-represented in ART programmes, data on viral suppression[2] shows variations by age among males who are HIV-positive (Simbayi et al., 2019). Among males, viral load (VL) suppression was the highest among HIV-positive people ages 50 and older (76.4%) and 45–49 years (71.8%). Similarly, among females, VL suppression was the highest among those aging 45–49 years (74.6%) and those ages 50 and older (71.2%). When males and females were compared across age groups (ages 0–14 years – males 56.1% and females 48%; 15–24 years – males 49.1% and females 47.0%; 45–49 year males), VL suppression was higher among males, except in the ages 25–34 years (males 41.5% and females 69.0%) and 45–49 years (males 71.8% and 75%, where it was higher among females). There is a need to investigate and understand sex differences, in particular why females and males in certain age groups show different rates of VL suppression (Simbayi et al., 2019).

---

[2]Viral load (VL) suppression is defined as a VL of <1000 copies HIV RNA/mL and is a measure of ART efficacy. It is used as a proxy indicator for adherence to treatment and for the risk of HIV transmission. A higher VL suppression means that treatment is effective.

The South African government has embarked extensive campaign to increase the uptake of HIV testing services (HTS) (NDoH 2016/2017). The 90–90–90[3] cascade also show sex differences in these key indicators with regard to HIV testing; a higher proportion of females than males knew their HIV status (88.9% vs 78.0%), were on ART (72.2% vs 67.4%), and had better VL suppression (89.9% vs 82.1%). In total 75.2% of participants indicated that they had ever tested for HIV in 2017. The highest number of people who had been tested in the previous 12 months were females (79.3%) (Simbayi et al., 2019). Previous studies have consistently shown lower rates of testing rates among males (Granich et al., 2008) which has been attributed to social norms that inform what it means to be a man and structural factors that inform men's health-seeking behaviour (Mfecane, 2018). Of concern in South Africa is that males aging 15 years and older were more likely to be unaware of having an HIV-positive status compared to their female counterparts. When all age and sex groups were compared, males aging 15–24 years were more likely to be unaware of their HIV-positive status, with 75.9% of HIV-positive men in this category unaware of their status compared to 36.2% of HIV-positive women in the same age group. However, women ages 50 and older were more likely to be unaware of their HIV-positive status, with 53.8% falling within this category compared to 45.4% of their male counterparts within the same age group. This again may be pointing to the role of targeting younger age groups for interventions and how this has a potential of leaving some populations out of the HIV response.

Earlier we have highlighted sex differences in key behavioural indicators, medical male circumcision (MMC), and gender-based violence, including aspects of gender norms that intersect to determine vulnerability. In conclusion, the previous section has underscored the need for a gender lens not only in research but policymaking and programme responses. Evidence shows that women, men, boys, and girls experience differential risk and vulnerability to HIV infection due to gender inequity as well as racism and socioeconomic-related inequity. There is also an urgent need to look closely at how targeting maybe leading to unintended consequences of leaving out of the response some portions of the population and also neglecting gender-focused intervention as a result of the emphasis on biomedical interventions. The case study had demonstrated the use of sex-disaggregated data not only to understand the epidemic but also to identify the gaps and also evaluate the intersection of men's issues and

---

[3] The 90–90–90 indicators are defined by UNAIDS as follows: the first 90 – the proportion of people living with HIV who know their HIV-positive status. In this study, people were classified as knowing their HIV-positive status if they reported that the last time they had an HIV test; they were informed that they were HIV-positive; or their blood sample (for this study) was confirmed as positive for ARV by a laboratory. The second 90 – the proportion of people who were on ART, as a subgroup of those who knew their HIV-positive status. Being on ART was defined as ART metabolites detected in the blood sample. The third 90 – the proportion who were virally suppressed among those who knew their HIV status and were on ART (as defined above).

those of women. The next goal is to increasingly integrate measures of gender, such as studies, and also, as encouraged by Clow et al. (2009), "to explore mechanisms for addressing the binary of male and female by developing measures of sex that are more nuanced and inclusive." This is being implemented for the 2021 SABSSM survey.

Integration of SGBA Research into Practice

The previous section has illustrated the importance of SGBA in tracking the response to the HIV epidemic in South Africa. However, it is clear that applying SGBA is a challenge as it goes beyond just the data surveys collect and requires more sensitive and nuanced measuring mechanisms. It has been stated that while SGBA can be challenging within the programme planning and the policy front, it is crucial for identifying and redressing gender inequities that create health disparities (Clow et al., 2009). If indeed one conceptualizes SGBA as a process, it stands to reason that one will need to adapt it in research, planning, and policy contexts. There is also a need to revisit and re-evaluate national policies and international guidelines using a SGBA lens. If research is designed with SGBA considerations, translation of the evidence into action will be more likely.

In conclusion, it remains imperative to glean lessons from countries that have made attempts to integrate SGBA in population health research or interventions in order to use evidence from research to improve health outcomes. Though the case studies in this chapter present evidence of the need for including sex and gender aggregated data where possible, as well as the need to translate the evidence into strategies or policies, there are some important final messages. Firstly, SGBA can be time-consuming (Theobald et al., 2017). A myriad of partnerships have to be brokered for negotiations of joint efforts, data ownership, buy-in, and consensus-building across stakeholders, and these may have different cultures and management approaches. Establishing and managing of sound and effective SGBA partnerships require an immense time investment.

As noted in this chapter, there is irrefutable evidence of the overlap and conflated definitions of sex and gender (Krieger, 2003) both in research and practice. Given this, there is an urgent need to build capacity within different institutional cultures not only to succinctly conceptualize the terms but also to build skills and capacity to design research with specific SGBA variables. Further, challenges were noted with regard to designing quantitative research that will specifically consider SGBA (Bowleg, 2012; Gottlieb, 1994; United Nations, 1995).

Several efforts are required to promote the translation of health outcome evidence into health policy in pragmatic terms. The ministries of health and relevant departments need to advocate for health information systems (HIS) that are inclusive of sex- and gender-disaggregated data. Having HIS that is SGBA compliant will open streams of resources that may be used to build skills in an array of issues as a conduit to promoting the translation of SGBA data into policy action. When translating research to practice, it is imperative to use trusted approaches and well-defined indicators. Also, the SABSSM in South Africa used research methodologies which are grounded in tested theories and trustworthy analysis creates the demand and use of findings. Indicators are crucial for tracking progress, and if properly defined, they can assist with the analysis of data. The indicators for gender disparity in health need to be further developed in order to measure social and structural determinants that can be linked to the impacts on the differential health outcomes of women, men and gender diverse populations (Sherwood et al., 2007).

The priority of government structures, donor interests, and involvement and nature of the evidence can influence whether or not research is translated into practice. On the other hand, the perception of policymakers regarding the strength and rigor of the SGBA evidence presented and backed by international recommendations is crucial. Finally, the active partnerships between research and policy actors are crucial, as well as links between researcher networks and policymakers, for facilitating knowledge transfer. This may potentially help to shape future strategies to bridge the research-policy gaps and ultimately improve the uptake of evidence in decision-making (Hutchinson et al., 2011).

In moving SGBA forward, there is a need for a multi-sectoral policy response to gender inequities in health promotion and disease prevention. This may include a joint commitment for policy through the development of objectives related to gender equity in health, the identification of health determinants, and the development of strategies to tackle contributing factors that affect health equity, and the documenting and disseminating of effective gender-sensitive policies to further facilitate learning across countries and regions (Ostlin et al., 2007).

References

Abrahams, N., Jewkes, R., & Mathews, S. (2010). Guns and gender-based violence in South Africa. *SAMJ: South African Medical Journal, 100*(9), 586–588.

Aulakh, A., & Anand, S. (2007). Sex and gender subgroup analyses of randomized trials. *Women's Health Issues, 17*(6), 342–350. https://doi.org/10.1016/j.whi.2007.04.002

Bird, C., & Rieker, P. (1999). Gender matters: An integrated model for understanding men's and women's health. *Social Sciences and Medicine, 48*(6), 745–755.

Bowleg, L. (2012). The problem with the phrase women and minorities: Intersectionality-an important theoretical framework for public health. *American Journal of Public Health, 102*(7), 1267–1273. https://doi.org/10.2105/AJPH.2012.300750

Campbell, A., Brooks, A., Pavlicova, M., Hu, M., Hatch-Maillette, M., Calsyn, D., & Tross, S. (2016). Barriers to condom use: Results for men and women enrolled in HIV risk reduction trials in outpatient drug treatment. *Journal of HIV/AIDS & Social Services, 15*(2), 130–146. https://doi.org/10.1080/15381501.2016.1166090

Canadian Institutes of Health Research. (2012). *IGH relevance review criteria.* http://www.cihr-irsc.gc.ca/e/45212.html

Clow, B., Pederson, A., Haworth-Brockman, M., & Bernier, J. (2009). *Rising to the challenge: Sex- and gender-based analysis for health planning, policy and research in Canada.* Halifax: Atlantic Centre of Excellence for Women's Health.

Connell, R. (1987). *Gender and power.* Stanford: Stanford University Press.

Courtenay, W. (2000). Constructions of masculinity and their influence on men's well-being: A theory of gender and health. *Social Science and Medicine, 50*(10), 1385–1401.

Day, S., Mason, R., Lagosky, S., & Rochon, P. (2016). Integrating and evaluating sex and gender in health research. *Health Research Policy and Systems, 14*(1). https://doi.org/10.1186/s12961-016-0147-7

Dellar, R. C., Dlamini, S., & Karim, Q. A. (2015). Adolescent girls and young women: Key populations for HIV epidemic control. *Journal of the International AIDS Society, 18*(2 Suppl 1), 19408.

De Oliveira, T., Kharsany, A., Gräf, T., Cawood, C., Khanyile, D., Grobler, A., Puren, A., Madurai, S., Baxter, C., Abdool, K., Karim, Q., & Karim, A. (2016). Transmission networks and risk of HIV infection in KwaZulu-Natal, South Africa: A community-wide phylogenetic study. *The Lancet HIV, 4.* https://doi.org/10.1016/S2352-3018(16)30186-2

Doyal, L. (2001). Informed consent: Moral necessity or illusion? *BMJ Quality & Safety, 10*, i29–i33.

Dunn, J., & Hayes, M. (1999). Toward a lexicon of population health. *Canada Journal of Public Health, 90*(suppl 1), S7–S10.

Evan, M., Risher, K., Zungu, N., Shisana, O., Moyo, S., Celentano, D. D., et al. (2016). Age-disparate sex and HIV risk for young women from 2002 to 2012 in South Africa. *Journal of the International AIDS Society, 19*(1), 21310. https://doi.org/10.7448/IAS.19.1.21310

Evans, T. M., Sing, D. K., Wakeford, H. R., Nikolov, N., Ballester, G. E., Drummond, B., Kataria, T., Gibson, N. P., Amundsen, D. S., & Spake, J. (2016). Detection of H_2O and evidence for TiO/VO in an ultra hot exoplanet atmosphere. *Astrophysical Journal Letter, 822*(1), L4. https://doi.org/10.3847/2041-8205/822/1/L4

Evans, M., Maughan-Brown, B., Zungu, N. P. and George, G. (2017). HIV prevalence and ART use among men in partnerships with 15-24 year old women in South Africa: HIV risk implications for young women in age-disparate partnerships. AIDS and Behavior. March 7 https://doi.org/10.1007/s10461-017-1741-6.

Federal, Provincial, & Territorial Advisory Committee on Population Health. (1994). Strategies for Population Health: Investing in the Health of Canadians.

Gaudet, S. (2007). *Emerging adulthood: A new stage in the life course. Implications for policy development.* Ottawa: Policy Research Initiative.

Gesensway, D. (2001). Reasons for sex-specific and gender-specific study of health topics. *Annals of Internal Medicine, 135*(10), 935. https://doi.org/10.7326/0003-4819-135-10-200111200-00032

Gourevitch, M. (2014). Population health and the academic medical center. *Academic Medicine, 89*(4), 544–549. https://doi.org/10.1097/acm.0000000000000171

Gottlieb, A. (1994). Saying good bye to health sharing. *Canada Women Studies, 14*(3), 117–118.

Gopalakrishnan, S., & Ganeshkumar, P. (2013). Systematic reviews and meta-analysis: Understanding the best evidence in primary healthcare. *Journal of Family Medicine and Primary Care, 2*(1), 9–14. https://doi.org/10.4103/2249-4863.109934

Granich, R., Gilks, C., Dye, C., De Cock, K., & Williams, B. (2008). Universal voluntary HIV testing with immediate antiretroviral therapy as a strategy for elimination of HIV transmission: A mathematical model. *Lancet.* https://doi.org/10.1016/S0140-6736(08)61697-9

Greaves et al. (1999). CIHR 2000: Sex, gender and women's health vancouver. *British Columbia Centre of Excellence in Women's Health.*

Greaves, L. (2011). Why put gender and sex into health research? In J. L. Oliffe & L. Greaves (Eds.), *Designing and conducting gender, sex and health research* (pp. 3–13). Thousand Oaks: Sage Publications, Inc..

Hankivsky, O., & Christoffersen, A. (2008). Intersectionality and the determinants of health: A Canadian perspective. *Critical Public Health, 18*(3), 271–283.

Hutchinson, E., Parkhurst, J., Phiri, S., Gibb, D., Chishinga, N., Droti, B., & Hoskins, S. (2011). National policy development for cotrimoxazole prophylaxis in Malawi, Uganda and Zambia: The relationship between Context, Evidence and Links. *Health Research Policy and Systems, 9*(S1). https://doi.org/10.1186/1478-4505-9-s1-s6

Health Canada. (2000). *Gender based analysis policy.* Ottawa: Available from www.hc sc.gc.ca/hl vs/women femmes/gender sexe/policypolitique eng.php.

Health Canada. (2003). Exploring concepts of gender and health Ottawa. *Women's Health Bureau.*

Heidari, S., Babor, T., De Castro, P., Trot, S., & Curno, M. (2016). Sex and gender equity in research: Rationale for SAGER guidelines and recommended use. *Research Integrity and Peer Review, 1*, 2.

Johnson, J., Greaves, L., & Repta, R. (2007). *Better science with sex and gender: A primer for Health Research.* Vancouver: Women's Health Research Network.

Johnson, J., Greaves, L., & Repta, R. (2009). Better science with sex and gender: Facilitating the use of a sex and gender-based analysis in health research. *International Journal for Equity in Health, 8*(1), 14. https://doi.org/10.1186/1475-9276-8-14

Johnson, J., & Beaude, A. (2013). Sex and gender reporting in health research: Why Canada should be a leader. *Canada Journal of Public Health, 104*(1), e80–e81.

Johnson LF, Dorrington RE & Moolla H (2017) Progress towards the 2020 targets for HIV diagnosis and antiretroviral treatment in South Africa. Southern African Journal of HIV Medicine 18(1):a694. https://doi.org/10.4102/sajhivmed.v18i1.694.

Kenyon CR, Tsoumanis A, Schwartz IS, Maughan-Brown B. (2016) Partner concurrency and HIV infection risk in South Africa. Int J Infect Dis. 45:81–7. https://doi.org/10.1016/j.ijid.2016.03.001.

Khayyam-Nekouei, Z., Neshatdoost, H., Yousefy, A., Sadeghi, M., & Manshaee, G. (2013). Psychological factors and coronary heart disease. *ARYA Atherosclerosis, 9*(1), 102–111.

Kindig, D., & Stoddart, G. (2003). What is population health? *American Journal of Public Health, 93*, 380–383. https://doi.org/10.2105/ajph.93.3.380

Krieger, N. (2003). Genders, sexes, and health: What are the connections—And why does it matter? *International Journal of Epidemiology, 32*(4), 652–657. https://doi.org/10.1093/ije/dyg156

Labonte, R., Schrecker, T., & Sen Gupta, A. (2005). *Health for some: Death, disease and disparity in a globalizing era.* Toronto: Centre for Social Justice Research and Education.

Lawrence, K., & Rieder, A. (2007). Methodologic and ethical ramifications of sex and gender differences in public health research. *Gender Medicine, 4*, S96–S105. https://doi.org/10.1016/s1550-8579(07)80050-7

Madiba S. & Ngwenya N. (2017) Cultural practices, gender inequality and inconsistent condom use increase vulnerability to HIV infection: narratives from married and cohabiting women in rural communities in Mpumalanga province, South Africa, Global Health Action, 10:sup2, 1341597. https://doi.org/10.1080/16549716.2017.1341597.

Martinez, G., & Abma, J. (2015). Sexual activity, contraceptive use, and childbearing of teenagers aged 15–19 in the United States. *NCHS Data Brief, 23*, 1–8.

Maughan-Brown, B., Evans, M., & George.G. (2016). Sexual behaviour of men and women within age-disparate partnerships in South Africa: Implications for young women's HIV risk. *PLoS One, 11*(8), e0159162.

Mayer, K., Bradford, J., Makadon, H., Stall, R., Goldhammer, H., & Landers, S. (2008). Sexual and gender minority health: What we know and what needs to be done. *American Journal of Public Health, 98*, 989–995. https://doi.org/10.2105/AJPH.2007.127811

Mfecane, S. (2018). Towards African-centred theories of masculinity. *Social Dynamics, 44*(2), 291–305. https://doi.org/10.1080/02533952.2018.1481683

Nowatzki, N., & Grant, K. (2010). Sex is not enough: The need for gender-based analysis in health research. *Health Care for Women International, 32*(4), 263–277. https://doi.org/10.1080/07399332.2010.519838

Ostlin, P., Eckermann, E., Mishra, U., Nkowane, M., & Wallstam, E. (2007). Health promotion challenges. Gender and health promotion: A multisectoral policy approach. *Health Promotion International, 21*(1), 25–35. https://doi.org/10.1093/heapro/dal048

Ovseiko, et al. (2016). A global call for action to include gender in research impact assessment. *Health Research Policy and Systems, 14*, 50.

Pan American Health Organization. (1999). Methodological summaries: Measuring inequity in health. *Epidemiology Bulletin, 20*(1).

Pines HA, Gorbach PM, Weiss RE, Reback CJ, Landovitz RJ, et al. (2016) Individual-level, partnership-level, and sexual event-level predictors of condom use during receptive anal inter-course among HIV-negative men who have sex with men in Los Angeles. AIDS and Behavior 20(6): 1315–1326. http://doi.org/10.1007/s10461-015-1218-4.

Pitpitan EV, Smith LR, Goodman-Meza D, Torres K, Semple SJ, et al. (2016) "Outness" as a mod-erator of the association between syndemic conditions and HIV risk-taking behaviour among men who have sex with men in Tijuana, Mexico. AIDS and Behavior 20(2):431–438.

Public Health Agency of Canada. (2001). *Towards a common understanding: Clarifying the core concepts of population health*. Retrieved on December 9, 2011, from http://www.phac-aspc.gc.ca/ph-sp/docs/common-commune/execsumm-eng.php

Public Health Agency of Canada. (2012). Chapter 2. The Chief Public Health Officer's Report on the State of Public Health in Canada– Sex, gender and public health.

Raphael, D. (2004). Social determinants of health, Canadian perspectives.

Richter, L., Mabaso, M., Ramjith, J., & Norris, S. (2015). Early sexual debut: Voluntary or coerced? Evidence from longitudinal data in South Africa – the Birth to Twenty Plus study. South African Medical Journal, [S.l.], v. 105, n. 4, p. 204–307, mar. 2015. ISSN 2078-5135.

Rider, G., McMorris, B., Gower, A., et al. (2018). Health and care utilization of transgender and gender nonconforming youth: A population-based study. *Pediatrics, 141*(3), e20171683.

Ruiz, M., & Verbrugge, L. (1997). A two way view of gender bias in medicine. *Journal of Epidemiology & Community Health, 51*(2), 106–109. https://doi.org/10.1136/jech.51.2.106

Runnels,V., Tudiver, S., Doull,M., & Boscoe, M. (2014). Challenges of including sex/gender anal-ysis in systematic reviews: a qualitative study, Systematic Review, 3:33

Seth, P., Lang, D. L., Diclemente, R. J., Braxton, N. D., Crosby, R. A., Brown, L. K., & Donenberg, G. R. (2012). Gender differences in sexual risk behaviours and sexually transmissible infec-tions among adolescents in mental health treatment. *Sexual Health, 9*(3), 240–246. https://doi.org/10.1071/SH10098

Sherwood, N., Adams, B., Isaac, E., Wu, S., & Fradinger, E. (2007). Knocked down and out: PACAP in development, reproduction and feeding. *Peptides, 28*(9), 1680–1687. https://doi.org/10.1016/j.peptides.2007.03.008

Shisana, O., & Simbayi, L. (2002). *Nelson Mandela/HSRC study of HIV/AIDS: South African national HIV prevalence, behavioural risks and mass media household survey 2002*. Cape Town: HSRC.

Shisana, O., Rehle, T., Simbayi, L. C., Zuma, K., Jooste, S., Pillay-Van Wyk, V., Mbelle, N., Van Zyl, J., Parker, W., Zungu, N. P., Pezi, S., & Implementation Team, S. A. B. S. S. M. I. I. I. (2009). *South African national HIV prevalence, incidence, behaviour and communication survey, 2008: Turning the tide among teenagers?* Cape Town: HSRC Press.

Shisana, O., Rehle, T., Simbayi, L. C., Parker, W., Zuma, K., Bhana, A., Connoly, C., Jooste, S., & Pillay, V. (2005). *South African national HIV prevalence, HIV incidence, behaviour and com-munication survey, 2005*. Cape Town: HSRC Press.

Shisana, O., Rehle, T., Simbayi, L. C., Zuma, K., Jooste, S., Zungu, N., Labadarios, D., Onoya, D., et al. (2014). *South African national HIV prevalence, incidence and behaviour survey, 2012*. Cape Town: HSRC Press.

Shisana O, Zungu N, Evans M, Risher K, Rehle T, Clementano D. (2015). The case for expand-ing the definition of 'key populations' to include high-risk groups in the general population to improve targeted HIV prevention efforts. S Afr Med J. 105(8):664-9. https://doi.org/10.7196/samjnew.7918. PMID: 26449696.

Simbayi, L.C., Zuma, K., Zungu, N., Moyo, S., Marinda, E., Jooste, S., Mabaso, M., Ramlagan, S., North, A., van Zyl, J., Mohlabane, N., Dietrich, C., Naidoo, I. and the SABSSMV Team (2019) South African National HIV Prevalence, Incidence, Behaviour and Communication Survey, 2017. Cape Town: HSRC Press.

Teich, N. (2012). Transgender 101: A simple guide to a complex issue. *Journal of Social Work, 13*(3), 333–334. https://doi.org/10.1177/1468017312457954

Theobald S, MacPherson EE, Dean L, et al 20 years of gender mainstreaming in health: lessons and reflections for the neglected tropical diseases community BMJ Global Health 2017;2:e000512.

UNAIDS (2014) 90–90–90 An ambitious treatment target to help end the AIDS epidemic. Geneva: UNAIDS.

UNAIDS (2015) Consultation on concurrent sexual partnerships: Recommendations from a meeting of the UNAIDS reference group on estimates, modelling and projection held in Nairobi Kenya. Updated November 2009. http://www.epidem.org/sites/default/files/reports/Concurrency_meeting_recommendations_Updated_Nov_2009.pdf.

United Nations. (1995). United Nations. Beijing declaration and platform for action. In *Fourth World Conference on Women*. Beijing.

UNAIDS. (2016). *Prevention among adolescent girls and young women: Putting HIV prevention Fast tracking*. Geneva: UNAIDS, Retrieved from https://www.unaids.org/sites/default/files/media_asset/UNAIDS_HIV_prevention_among_adolescent_girls_and_young_women.pdf.

UNAIDS. (2019). *UNAIDS data 2019*. Geneva: UNAIDS. Retrieved from https://www.unaids.org/sites/default/files/media_asset/2019-UNAIDS-data_en.pdf

UNICEF. (2011). Gender influences on child survival, health and nutrition: A narrative review. Retrieved from https://www.unicef.org/Gender_Influences_on_Child_Survival_a_Narrative_review.pdf.

Visser, M., Makin, J., Vandormael, A., Sikkema, K., & Forsyth, B. (2009). HIV/AIDS stigma in a South African community. *AIDS Care, 21*(2), 197–206. https://doi.org/10.1080/09540120801932157

Vlassoff, C., & Moreno, C. (2002). Placing gender at the centre of health programming: Challenges and limitations. *Social Science & Medicine, 54*(11), 1713–1723. https://doi.org/10.1016/s0277-9536(01)00339-2

Part II
SGBA Matters

Chapter 4
HIV Prevention and the Need for Gender-Transformative Approaches

Jacqueline Gahagan and Shari L. Dworkin

Introduction

This chapter examines the issues associated with the early epidemiology of HIV, the AIDS risk and vulnerability paradigms and how these have served to overlook populations of cisgender and transgender women and heterosexual men in public health HIV prevention responses in North America. In this chapter we argue that notions of HIV sexual risk-taking and the overarching absence of heterosexually identified cisgender and transgender women and heterosexual men from early HIV public health interventions and clinical trials served to further the gender-blind approach whereby HIV risk-taking was regarded as being associated with gay male identity and that as a consequence other populations were not seen to be at risk. Further, we argue that the use of the terms sex and gender interchangeably in HIV-related public health and clinical interventions was and continues to be problematic in understanding the unique physiological and gendered elements associated with HIV infection (Gahagan et al., 2015). For example, the use of single-sex, cisgender male-only HIV clinical trial data to determine HIV RNA levels as the de facto measure for the initiation of antiretroviral therapy (ART) and the subsequent extrapolation of pharmacokinetics and effectiveness data on ART to women were problematic (Gahagan & Loppie, 2003). Further, the lack of reference to and framing of the gender-related social determinants contributing to differential HIV infection rates, access to and uptake of HIV testing, HIV treatment adherence, access to and use of pre-exposure prophylaxis (PrEP), issues of HIV disclosure, gender-based violence, among others, served to limit our

J. Gahagan (✉)
Faculty of Health, Dalhousie University, Halifax, NS, Canada
e-mail: jgahagan@dal.ca

S. L. Dworkin
School of Nursing and Health Studies, University of Washington Bothell, Bothell, WA, USA

© Springer Nature Switzerland AG 2021
J. Gahagan, M. K. Bryson (eds.), *Sex- and Gender-Based Analysis in Public Health*, https://doi.org/10.1007/978-3-030-71929-6_4

understanding of the pandemic among other diverse populations (Campbell, 1995; Dworkin et al., 2009; Dworkin & Ehrhardt, 2007). Our chapter concludes with a discussion on the need for gender-transformative approaches to HIV and AIDS prevention, treatment, and support in public health, particularly in relation to addressing the enduring disparities in access to and uptake of public health interventions aimed at reducing the burden of HIV in the North American context.

Background

While HIV continues to represent an enduring public health challenge globally, in the North American context, it was initially framed as a disease affecting only gay men, hence limiting our understanding of the gendered nature of the epidemic particularly in relation to, for example, heterosexual transmission. The initial naming of HIV as gay-related immune deficiency or GRID in the early 1980s and the overall limited public health response toward gay men impacted by HIV who were seen as the primary "at-risk" population in both the United States and Canada was problematic and had long-standing implications for HIV prevention efforts (Dworkin, 2015; Dworkin & Ehrhardt, 2007; Gahagan et al., 2013). In addition, early HIV biomedical and clinical research linked to the progression of HIV symptoms and to opportunistic infections such as Kaposi sarcoma or "gay cancers", among other infections, signalled a diagnosis of acquired immune deficiency syndrome or AIDS. In the face of no effective treatments or cures, a diagnosis of AIDS was regarded as a certain death sentence in the early years of the epidemic. While the scientific research evidence on the relationship between HIV and AIDS became clearer, what was less clear was how this mounting evidence base would inform efforts for a coordinated national scaling-up of public health responses to HIV prevention among gay men and other populations in North America. What emerged in response to the perceived lack of timely government action to a major public health threat was the coordinated efforts among gay men to develop community-based initiatives to mobilize governments for greater investment in research at a time when there were essentially no available treatments. The resultant HIV and AIDS activism was aimed at pushing governments for greater investment in scientific research to prevent the spread of the virus and to develop effective treatments for those living with an HIV or AIDS diagnosis.

The rise of a highly organized HIV and AIDS social movement in North America in the early 1980s, including the Gay Men's Health Crisis in New York City and the AIDS Committee of Toronto, among others, played an instrumental role in leveraging support for HIV- and AIDS-targeted research funding particularly in basic, clinical, and public health fields (Kayal, 1993; Stockdale, 1993). As community mobilization grew, so too did the push for public health to scale up HIV prevention interventions to address the contested "risk group" debates and prevention messages in the face of growing epidemiological evidence being presented at national and international HIV and AIDS conferences indicating the impact of the pandemic was more widespread than originally conceptualized. In 1983 at a satellite AIDS forum, The Denver Principles were developed to ensure gay men living with HIV or AIDS were involved in every level of decision-making at both a personal and a healthcare system level. At the same time, the slow public health and clinical shift toward other populations impacted by HIV such as intravenous drug users (who were contracting the virus through used syringes and other drug paraphernalia), sex workers (who were becoming infected through unprotected sex with their clients and partners), and to a lesser degree pregnant women (in terms of vertical transmission from the pregnant woman to the fetus) who were being diagnosed in greater numbers and which required a rethinking of public health HIV "risk group" messaging. Missing from these early public health prevention efforts was the discussion of how and why a sex- and gender-based analysis would offer greater clarity in furthering our understanding of key social and biological drivers of the epidemic and in developing gender-transformative responses to combatting the increasing infections rates among, for example, both cisgender and transgender women who were contracting HIV in the early years of the epidemic (Bockting et al., 2005; Dworkin, 2005; Rao Gupta, 2001).

However, despite this general lack of sex- and gender-based analysis, a significant shift in public health messaging related to HIV risk began to emerge from the growing body of epidemiological data indicating, for example, increased infection rates among newborns due to vertical transmission from previously undiagnosed women to the fetus (Gahagan et al., 2013; Leonard et al., 2001; Rao Gupta, 2001). In addition, there was a growing trend of women – often women of colour - living in poverty, seeking HIV assistance and who were ill but could not access housing or disability resources allotted to HIV-positive people given that they could not gain access to an HIV/AIDS diagnosis (Watkins-Hayes, 2019). Eventually, lawyers had to file a class action lawsuit against the Department of Health and Human Services in order to change the US Centers for Disease Control (CDC) case definition to include common disease manifestations among cisgender women such as invasive cervical cancer and recurrent yeast infections (Exner et al., 1999). Of importance, the original HIV case definition also omitted bacterial pneumonia and tuberculosis from its boundaries, thus excluding a large population of women, and particularly the growing number of women of colour experiencing poverty and racism (Watkins-Hayes, 2019). In 1993, the CDC case definition was changed to include 'female-specific' presentations of the virus which in turn led to an explosive increase in women being rendered visible in the US epidemic (Dworkin, 2005; Exner et al., 1999; Watkins-Hayes, 2019).

Once the CDC case definition was changed, the cases of women with AIDS in the United States increased from 6% in 1984 to 19% in 1995. Along with this growth in numbers came the recognition that there was an increasing proportion of cases attributable to heterosexual transmission. In 1994 in the US, heterosexual contact surpassed intravenous drug use as the predominant route of transmission among women with a diagnosis of AIDS (CDC, 1995), and HIV infection became the third leading cause of death among women aged 25–44, followed by cancer and unintentional injuries (Centers for Disease Control, 1996). By the mid-1990s, there was no longer any doubt that HIV had become a major public health problem for women in the United States. Further, it also was clear that the epidemic was striking the poorest and most marginalized women, many of whom lived in inner cities in the Eastern United States (Exner et al., 2003; Watkins-Hayes, 2019). Racialized trends continue today with 57% of new HIV infections found among African American women, 18% among Hispanic/Latina women, and 21% among White women (CDC, 2018).

In the Canadian context, the disproportionate burden of HIV has also been among gay men; however, the proportion of gay men had varied over time while the rates of HIV diagnoses among females increased. According to 2018 surveillance data, the majority (64%) of reported HIV cases among Canadian females are attributed to the heterosexual exposure category. In terms of the proportion of reported HIV cases by age among Canadian females in general, those between the ages of 30 and 39 had the highest proportion of new HIV diagnoses at 34%, followed by females 40–49 at 23%, 22% for females 50 years of age and over, 17% for females between 20 and 29, and 2% for those between 15 and 19, as is the case for females under the age of 15 years (Haddad et al., 2019). It is noteworthy that such increases in reported HIV cases among females in Canada have not been reported in many other high-income countries. It is also important to note that the collection of national HIV data for race/ethnicity is varied in Canada but that Indigenous populations are overrepresented in HIV data where these data do exist (PHAC, 2016).

Why Sex and Gender Matter in HIV

Biological susceptibility to HIV, the gendered nature of HIV transmission, and the physiological response to treatment for HIV and sexually transmitted and blood-borne infections (STBBIs) more broadly suggest the need for greater attention to the sex and gender-based analysis of HIV infection (Ehrhardt et al., 1992). Early on in the HIV epidemic in North America, heterosexual women, including transgender women, were not regarded as "at risk" for HIV and were largely absent from HIV-specific public health interventions and community-based responses focused primarily on gay men (Arthur et al., 2013; Dworkin et al., 2009). Differences in treatment success with antiretroviral therapy where women were historically excluded from clinical trials resulted in challenges with adherence and poorer health outcomes for women living with HIV (Gahagan & Loppie, 2003). Where women were the focus of public health HIV prevention campaigns, it was often in relation to women being regarded as potential "vectors of disease" to children and as such, they were included largely in relation to the prevention of vertical transmission in the context of prenatal care practices. These campaigns stressed the importance of HIV testing as a normative part of prenatal care without addressing other intersecting determinants of health for expectant mothers such as income, geography, racism and ethnicity, poverty, gender-based volence, or housing, among others. In addition, women were intitially focused on as "vectors of disease" in relation to sex work with the resultant framing of HIV awareness campaigns in relation to the threat of transmitting HIV to the general population. Both preganant women and sex workers were viewed as secondary to fetuses and male clients who were viewed as the "real" victims of heterosexual HIV infection (Higgins et al., 2010).

It took vastly longer for evidence-based researchers and policy makers to design and implement gender-specific HIV prevention interventions that took cisgender women's gender-related risks into account. Early interventions at the time were often gender-neutral and relied on public health models of individual behavioural change such as the health belief model or the theory of reasoned action (Exner et al., 2003). These interventions were later critiqued for omitting the gendered risks women experience in their daily lives and relationships, their economic dependency on men, their experiences with gender-based violence, and their unique structural drivers of risk, such as poverty, racism and unstable housing (Drake & Gahagan, 2015; Dworkin & Ehrhardt, 2007; Krishnan et al., 2008; Rao Gupta et al., 2008). The main HIV prevention approach at that time was to encourage women to use male condoms which failed to note that male condoms needed to be negotiated in terms of use with an intimate male partner. A large body of HIV research then revealed how gendered power relations between women and men impeded women's negotiating power in sexual interactions and specifically in HIV prevention (Campbell, 1995; Ehrhardt et al., 1992; Ehrhardt & Exner, 2000; O'Leary, 2000), and thus it was necessary for interventions to become "gender-sensitive" to recognize the unique context of women's relationships and their experiences of gendered power relations along with desires for intimacy and trust (Amaro & Raj, 2000; Dworkin, 2006; Higgins et al., 2010; O'Leary, 2000). In addition, the gendered nature of sexual interactions themselves was identified as helping to drive HIV risks for women, whereby women were assumed to be socialized as "passive," other-oriented, and focused on male pleasure in sexual interactions, thereby negating their own needs in favour of "responsiveness" to men in sexual intimacy (Dworkin et al., 2007; Dworkin et al., 2009; Ehrhardt et al., 2000). Simultaneously, gendered sexual scripts for heterosexually active men lead many to be socialized to be sexually assertive and knowledgeable about sex; to have a right of access to women's bodies for sex in terms of timing, frequency, and fertility; and to see women as responsible for accommodating their sex drive with a focus on male pleasure (Dworkin & O'Sullivan, 2005; Rao Gupta, 2001; Seal & Ehrhardt, 2003).

Behavioural interventions that were "gender-sensitive" (sensitive to the gendered needs of women and men) and "gender-empowering" (challenging gender-based violence and harmful gender norms and/or reshaping the context in which safer sex decisions are made) were then born (Rao Gupta, 2001) and grew rapidly (Ehrhardt & Exner, 2000; Jemmot et al., 2007; Melendez et al., 2003; Sherman et al., 2006; Wingood et al., 2004). Similarly, a suite of primary prevention interventions were designed to inflect gender-based content to meet the needs of African American and other raciliazed women, highlighting how "gender-specific" or "race-specific" behavioural interventions may need to take into account the issue of intersectionality or the ways that multiple axes of identity and inequality simultaneously shape women's HIV risks and the realities of living with HIV (Berger, 2004; Ehrhardt & Exner, 2000; Gentry et al., 2005; Millett et al., 2007; Lyles et al., 2007; Rao Gupta et al., 2008; Watkins-Hayes, 2014; Wingood & DiClemente, 2006).

Following these efforts, women living with HIV in North America then received greater attention in interventions beyond primary prevention. However, it is important to note that women living with HIV are far more likely to have experienced violence and trauma than HIV-negative women and men who have enacted violence are far more likely to be HIV positive than men who have not enacted violence (Maman et al., 2002; O'Leary, 2000; Rigby & Johnson, 2017; Sareen et al., 2009). It is also the case that many women living with HIV experience cumulative trauma, violence, PTSD, and structural inequalities that not only serve to drive HIV risk but also in relation to health outcomes in HIV treatment and care (Berger, 2004). This has led to healthcare approaches that call for interventions that focus on trauma-informed perspectives with women living with HIV to help improve their HIV testing, treatment adherence, and other treatment-related outcomes (Cuca et al., 2019; Dawson-Rose et al., 2019; Machingter et al., 2019; Machtinger, Haberer, Wilson, et al., 2012; Machtinger, Haberer, Wilson, & Weiss, 2012). Similar findings concerning violence and trauma have also been documented among transgender women, highlighting the need to continually expand upon public health definitions of sex and gender and their interrelationship in order to design effective HIV prevention, care, and treatment interventions (Herbst et al., 2008; Melendez et al., 2006; Newmann et al., 2017; Poteat et al., 2014).

Equally troubling is the absence of public health messaging and the late recognition of the gendered prevention intervention needs of heterosexually active men who are HIV-negative as well as those who are living with HIV (Bowleg et al., 2011; Bowleg & Raj, 2012; Elwy et al., 2002). While it has been assumed that HIV among heterosexual men is linked to a bridge with bisexuality or with "on the down low," the stigma and prejudice associated with HIV can result in furthering the perception of HIV as a disease that largely or only impacts gay men (Dodge et al., 2008; Dworkin, 2015). However, research has now linked dominant notions of heterosexual masculinities (societal ideals about what it means to be a 'real man') to HIV risk and to HIV prevention, treatment, and care, including the role of masculinities in HIV testing behaviours and retention in the HIV treatment cascade (Barker et al., 2010; Dworkin et al., 2013; Dworkin, 2015; Exner et al., 1999; Fleming & Dworkin, 2015; Sileo et al., 2018). Among Black men in the US, data indicate a significant level of heterosexual transmission (Raj & Bowleg, 2012). In their seminal piece, Raj and Bowleg (2012) highlight a call to action given the recognition by the US CDC of the heightened risk of HIV that heterosexually active Black men and women face in the US and a "generalized epidemic" in these populations (CDC, 2009; CDC, 2011). Since that time, researchers have designed and implemented new gender- and race-sensitive approaches for Black heterosexually active men in the US that focus on structural (work-related) and social and interpersonal dimensions of masculinities (Raj et al., 2014; Raj et al., 2019). However, gender-transformative HIV prevention, treatment, and care interventions are vastly more common outside of the US and Canada and may not focus on structural drivers of HIV, reverting to more of a gender-equitable and gender-norm based approaches (Barker et al., 2010; Dworkin et al., 2015). Still, these approaches have been found to be promising in terms of significant improvements in reducing violence and HIV-related outcomes, along with improving several sexual and reproductive health outcomes (Casey et al., 2018; Dworkin et al., 2013; Ruane-McAteer et al., 2019) and could be increasingly applied to the North American context if successfully modified and scaled up.

Conclusion

It is noteworthy that the HIV and AIDS movement in North America, particularly among gay men, served as a catalyst for public health actions on issues of HIV prevention, treatment, and support in the early years of the pandemic. However, it was not until the threat of a generalized heterosexual epidemic and the resultant human rights battles that greater attention was brought to the interrogation of the intersecting issues of sex, gender and HIV prevention. Through advocacy by and for women, including those living with HIV, along with prevention campaigns to reduce vertical transmission, came a shift away from the initial at-risk paradigm associated with gay male populations. Both sex and gender continue to feature significantly in framing our gender-transformative understanding of the social contexts of health outcomes, from the gendered social expectations of HIV risk and health-seeking behaviours that can contribute to HIV-related health outcomes, as well as the ways in which biological sex can impact treatment success, including differences in pharmacokinetics. Yet the need remains for greater attention to gender-transformative approaches in public health HIV prevention, care, and treatment, and these approaches must continue to be the focus of addressing the epidemic in North America.

References

Amaro, H., & Raj, A. (2000). On the margin: Power and women's HIV risk reduction strategies. *Sex Roles, 42*, 723–749.

Arthur, J., Gahagan, J., Guay, J., & Beausoliel, K. (2013). Enhanced surveillance of women and HIV. In J. Gahagan (Ed.), *Women and HIV prevention in Canada*. Toronto, ON: Canadian Scholars' Press.

Barker, G., Ricardo, C., Nascimento, M., Olukoya, A., & Santos, C. (2010). Questioning gender norms with men to improve health outcomes: Evidence of impact. *Global Public Health, 5*, 539–553.

Berger, M. (2004). *Workable sisterhood: The political journey of stigmatized women with HIV*. Princeton: Princeton University Press.

Bockting, W. O., Robinson, B. E., Forberg, J., & Scheltema, K. (2005). Evaluation of a sexual health approach to reducing HIV/STD risk in the transgender community. *AIDS Care, 17*, 289–303.

Bowleg, et al. (2011). "What does it take to be a man? What is a real man?" Ideologies of masculinity and HIV sexual risk among Black heterosexual men. *Culture, Health and Sexuality, 13*, 545–559.

Bowleg, L., & Raj, A. (2012). Shared communities, structural contexts, and HIV risk: Prioritizing the HIV risk and prevention needs of Black heterosexual men. *American Journal of Public Health, 102*, S173–S177.

Campbell, C. (1995). Male gender roles and sexuality: Implications for women's AIDS risk and prevention. *Social Science and Medicine, 41*, 97–210.

Casey, E., Carlson, J., Two, B. S., et al. (2018). Gender transformative approaches to engaging men in gender-based violence prevention: A review and conceptual model. *Trauma, Violence, and Abuse, 19*(2), 231–246.

CDC (1995). https://www.cdc.gov/mmwr/preview/mmwrhtml/00039622.htm

Centers for Disease Control. (2018). *Diagnosis of HIV Infection in the United States.* Available at: https://www.cdc.gov/hiv/pdf/library/reports/surveillance/cdc-hiv-surveillance-report-2018-preliminary-vol-30.pdf

Centers for Disease Control and Prevention. (2009). *The heightened national response to the HIV/ AIDS crisis among African Americans.* Available at: http://www.cdc.gov/hiv/topics/aa/cdc.htm

Centers for Disease Control and Prevention (CDC). (1996). Update: Mortality attributableto HIV infection among persons aged 25–44 years–United States, 1994. *Morbidity Mortality Weekly Report, 45*, 121–125.

Centers for Disease Control and Prevention. (2011). Disparities in diagnoses of HIV infection between Blacks/African Americans and other racial/ethnic populations—37 states, 2005–CDC Health Disparities and Inequalities Report—United States, 2011. *Morbidity Mortality Weekly Report, 60*, 93–98.

Cuca, Y. P., Shumway, M., Machinger, E. L., Davis, K., Khanna, N., Cocohoba, J., & Dawson-Rose, C. (2019). The association of trauma with the physical, behavioural and social health of women living with HIV: Pathways to guide trauma-informed health care interventions. *Women's Health Issues, 29*, 276–284.

Dawson-Rose, C., Cuca, Y. P., Shumway, M., Davis, K., & Machinger, E. L. (2019). Providing primary care for HIV in the context of trauma: Experiences of the health care team. *Women's Health Issues, 29*, 385–391.

Dodge, B., Jeffries, W. L., & Sanford, T. G. M. (2008). Beyond the Down Low: Sexual risk, protection and disclosure among at risk men who have sex with women and men (MSMW). *Archives of Sexual Behavior, 37*, 683–696.

Drake, C., & Gahagan, J. (2015). Working "upstream": Why we shouldn't use heterosexual women as health promotion change agents in HIV-prevention interventions aimed at heterosexual men. *Health Care for Women International, 26*(11), 1270–1289. https://doi.org/10.1080/0739933 2.2015.1005305

Dworkin, S. L. (2006). Revisiting "success:" post-trial analysis of a gender-specific HIV prevention intervention. *AIDS and Behavior, 10*, 41–51.

Dworkin, S. L. (2005). Who is epidemiologically fathomable in the HIV/AIDS epidemic? Gender, sexuality, and intersectionality in public health. *Culture, Health, and Sexuality, 7*, 16–23.

Dworkin, S. L., & O'Sullivan, L. (2005). Actual vs desired initiation patterns among a sample of college-aged men: Tapping disjunctures within traditional male sexual scripts. *Journal of Sex Research, 42*, 150–158.

Dworkin, S. L., & Ehrhardt, A. A. (2007). Going beyond ABC to include GEM (gender relations, economic contexts, and migration movements): Critical reflections on progress in the HIV/ AIDS epidemic. *American Journal of Public Health, 97*, 13–16.

Dworkin, S. L., Beckford, S. T., & Ehrhardt, A. A. (2007). Sexual scripts of women: A longitudinal analysis of participants in a gender-specific HIV prevention intervention. *Archives of Sexual Behavior, 36*, 269–279.

Dworkin, S. L., Fullilove, R., & Peacock, D. (2009). Are HIV/AIDS prevention interventions for heterosexually active men gender-specific? *American Journal of Public Health, 99*, 981–984.

Dworkin, S. L., Treves-Kagan, S., & Lippman, S. A. (2013). Gender-transformative interventions to reduce HIV risks and violence with heterosexually active men: A review of the global evidence. *AIDS and Behavior, 17*, 2845–2863.

Dworkin, S. L., Colvin, C., & Fleming, P. (2015). The promises and limitations of gender transformative health programming with men. *Culture, Health, and Sexuality, 17*, 128–143. https://doi.org/10.1080/13691058.2015.1035751

Dworkin, S. L. (2015). *Men at Risk: Masculinities, heterosexuality and HIV Prevention*. New York: NYU Press.

Ehrhardt, A. A., Exner, T. M., Hoffman, S., Siberman, I., Yingling, S., Adams-Skinner, J., & Smart-Smith, L. (2000). HIV//STD risk and sexual strategies among women family planning clients in New York: Project FIO. *AIDS and Behavior, 6*, 1–13.

Ehrhardt, A. A., & Exner, T. M. (2000). Prevention of sexual risk behavior for HIV infection with women. *AIDS, 14*, S53–S58.

Ehrhardt, A. A., Yingling, S., Zawadski, E., & Martinez-Ramirez, M. (1992). Prevention of heterosexual transmission of HIV: Barriers for women. *Journal of Psychology and Human Sexuality, 5*, 37–67.

Elwy, A. R., Hart, G. J., Hawkes, S., & Petticrew, M. (2002). Effectiveness of interventions to prevent sexually transmitted infections and human immunodeficiency virus in heterosexual men: A systematic review. *Archives of Internal Medicine, 162*, 1818–1830.

Exner, T. M., Hoffman, S., Dworkin, S. L., & Ehrhardt, A. A. (2003). Beyond the male condom: The evolution of gender-specific HIV interventions for women. *Annual Review of Sex Research, 14*, 114–136.

Exner, T. M., Gardos, P. S., Seal, D. W., & Ehrhardt, A. A. (1999). HIV sexual risk reduction interventions with heterosexual men: The forgotten group. *AIDS and Behavior, 3*, 347–358.

Fleming, P., & Dworkin, S. L. (2015). The importance of masculinity and gender norms for understanding institutional responses to HIV testing and treatment strategies. *AIDS, 30*, 157–158.

Gahagan, J., Gray, K., & Whynacht, A. (2015). Sex and gender matter in health research: addressing health inequities in health research reporting. *International Journal for Equity in Health, 14*, 12. https://doi.org/10.1186/s12939-015-0144-4

Gahagan, J., Ricci, C., Jackson, R., Prentice, T., Mill, J., & Adam, B. (2013). Advancing our knowledge: Findings of a meta-ethnographic synthesis. In J. Gahagan (Ed.), *Women and HIV prevention in Canada*. Toronto, ON: Canadian Scholars' Press.

Gahagan, J., & Loppie, C. (2003). Adherence to antiretroviral therapy among HIV+ women in Canada. In J. Lévy (Ed.), *Les multitherapies: Expériences et répercussions*. Quebec City, QU: Presses de l'université du Quebec.

Gentry, Q. M., Elifson, K., & Sterk, C. (2005). Aiming for more relevant HIV risk reduction: A Black feminist perspective for enhancing HIV prevention for low-income African American women. *AIDS Education and Prevention, 17*, 238–252.

Haddad, N., Robert, A., Weeks, A., Popovic, N., Siu, W., & Archibald, C. (2019). HIV in Canada – Surveillance report, 2018. *Canada Communicable Disease Report, 45*, 304–312.

Herbst, J.H., Jacobs, E.D., Finlayson, T.J. et al. Estimating HIV Prevalence and Risk Behaviors of Transgender Persons in the United States: A Systematic Review. AIDS Behav 12, 1–17 (2008). https://doi.org/10.1007/s10461-007-9299-3

Higgins, J. A., Hoffman, S., & Dworkin, S. L. (2010). Rethinking gender, heterosexual men, and women's vulnerability to HIV. *American Journal of Public Health, 100*, 435–445.

Jemmot, L. S., Jemmot, J. B., & O'Leary, A. (2007). Effects on sexual risk behavior of brief HIV/STD prevention interventions for African American women in primary care settings. *American Journal of Public Health, 97*, 1034–1040.

Kayal, P. M. (1993). *Bearing witness: Gay Men's health crisis and the politics of AIDS*. Westview Press.

Krishnan, S., Dunbar, M. S., Minnis, A. M., Medlin, C. A., Gerdts, C. E., & Padian, N. S. (2008). Poverty, gender inequities, and women's risk of human immunodeficiency virus/AIDS. *Annals of the New York Academy of Science, 1136*, 101–110.

O'Leary, A. (2000). Women at risk for HIV from a primary partner: Balancing risk and intimacy. *Annual Review of Sex Research, 11*, 191–234.

Leonard, L., Gahagan, J., Doherty, M. A., & Hankins, C. (2001). HIV Counseling and testing among pregnant women in Canada. In C. Amaratunga et al. (Eds.), *Gender, health, and HIV/AIDS: A reference manual for governments and other stakeholders*. United Kingdom, Commonwealth Secretariat.

Lyles, C.M., Kay, L.S., Crepaz, N., Herbst, J.H., Passin, W.F., Kim, A.S., Rama, S.M., Thadiparthi, S., DeLuca, J.B., & Mullins, M.M. (2007). HIV/AIDS Prevention Research Synthesis Team. Best-evidence interventions: findings from a systematic review of HIV behavioral interventions for US populations at high risk, 2000–2004. Am J Public Health. 97(1):133-43. https://doi.org/10.2105/AJPH.2005.076182. Epub 2006 Nov 30. PMID: 17138920; PMCID: PMC1716236.

Machingter, E. L., Davis, K. B., Kimberg, L. S., et al. (2019). From treatment to healing: Inquiry and response to recent past trauma in adult health care. *Women's Health Issues, 29*, 97–102.

Machtinger, E. L., Haberer, J. E., Wilson, T. C., & Weiss, D. S. (2012). Psychological trauma and PTSD in HIV-positive women: A meta-analysis. *AIDS and Behavior, 16*, 2091–2100.

Machtinger, E. L., Haberer, J. E., Wilson, T. C., et al. (2012). Recent trauma is associated with antiretroviral failure and HIV transmission risk behavior among HIV-positive women and female-identified transgenders. *AIDS and Behavior, 16*, 2160–2170.

Maman, S., Mbwambo, J. K., Hogan, N. M., Kilonzo, G. P., Campbell, J. D., Weiss, E., et al. (2002). HIV-positive women report more lifetime partner violence: Findings from a voluntary counselling and testing clinic in Dar es Salaam, Tanzania. *American Journal of Public Health, 92*, 1331–1337.

Melendez, R. M., Hoffman, S., Exner, T., Leu, C.-S., & Ehrhardt, A. A. (2003). Intimate partner violence and safer sex negotiation: Effects of a gender-specific intervention. *Archives of Sexual Behavior, 32*, 499–511.

Melendez, R. M., Bonem, L. A., & Sember, R. (2006). On bodies and research: Transgender issues in health and HIV research. *Sexuality Research and Social Policy, 3*, 21–38.

Millett, G. A, Flores, S. A, Peterson, J. L., & Bakeman, R. (2007). Explaining disparities in HIV infection among black and white men who have sex with men: a meta-analysis of HIV risk behaviors. AIDS. 1;21(15):2083–91. https://doi.org/10.1097/QAD.0b013e3282e9a64b. PMID: 17885299.

Newmann, M. S., Finlayson, T. J., Pitts, N. L., & Keatley, J. (2017). Comprehensive HIV prevention for transgender persons. *American Journal of Public Health, 107*, 207–212.

Poteat, T., Reisner, S., & Raddix, A. (2014). HIV epidemics among transgender women. *Current Opinion in HIV/AIDS, 9*, 168–173.

Public Health Agency of Canada. *HIV in Canada: Surveillance Report 2018 and the Summary: Estimates of HIV incidence, prevalence, and Canada's Progress on Meeting the 90–90-90 HIV target,* 2016 published by the Public Health Agency of Canada (PHAC).

Rao Gupta, G. (2001). Gender, sexuality, and HIV/AIDS: The what, the why, and the how. *SIECUS Report, 29*, 6–12.

Rao Gupta, G., Parkhurst, J. O., Ogden, J. A., Aggleton, P., & Mahal, A. (2008). Structural approaches to HIV prevention. *Lancet, 372*, 764–775.

Raj, A., & Bowleg, L. (2012). Heterosexual risk of HIV among Black men in the United States: A call to action against a neglected crisis in Black communities. *American Journal of Men's Health, 6*, 178–181.

Raj, A., Dasgupta, A., Goldson, I., Lafontant, D., Freeman, E., & Silverman, J. G. (2014). Pilot evaluation of the Making Employment Needs [MEN] count intervention: Addressing behavioral and structural HIV risks in heterosexual black men. *AIDS Care, 26*, 152–159.

Raj, A., Johns, N. E., Valida, F., et al. (2019). Evaluation of making employment needs count (MEN) intervention to reduce HIV/STI risk for Black heterosexual men in Washington DC. *American Journal of Men's Health, 13*. https://doi.org/10.1177/1557988319869493

Rigby, S. W., & Johnson, L.F., (2017). The relationship between intimate partner violence and HIV: A model-based evaluation. Infect Dis Model. 16;2(1):71–89. https://doi.org/10.1016/j.idm.2017.02.002. PMID: 29928730; PMCID: PMC5963327.

Ruane-McAteer, E., Amin, A., Hanratty, J., et al. (2019). Interventions addressing men, masculinities and gender equality in sexual and reproductive health and rights: An evidence and gap map and systematic review of reviews. *BMJ Global Health, 4*, e001634.

Sareen, J., Pagura, J., & Grant, B. (2009). Is intimate partner violence associated with HIV infection among women in the United States? *General Hospital Psychiatry, 31*, 274–278.

Seal, D., & Ehrhardt, A. A. (2003). Masculinity and urban men: Perceived scripts for courtship, romantic and sexual interactions with women. *Culture, Health and Sexuality, 5*, 295–319.

Sherman, S. G., German, Y., Cheng, M., Marks, M., & Bailey-Kloche, M. (2006). The evaluation of the JEWEL project: An innovative economic-enhancement and HIV-prevention intervention study targeting drug-using women involved in prostitution. *AIDS Care, 18*, 1–11.

Sileo, K., Fielding-Miller, R., Dworkin, S. L., & Fleming, P. (2018). What role do masculine norms play in Men's HIV testing in sub-Saharan Africa? A scoping review. *AIDS and Behavior, 22*, 2468–2479. https://doi.org/10.1007/s10461-018-2160-z

Stockdale, B. (1993). *Activism against AIDS: At the intersection of sexuality, race, gender.* Class: Lynne Reiner Publishers.

Watkins-Hayes, C. (2014). Intersectionality and the Sociology of HIV/AIDS: Past, present and future research directions. *Annual Review of Sociology, 40*, 431–457.

Watkins-Hayes, C. (2019). *Remaking a life: How women living with HIV/AIDS confront inequality.* Oakland: University of California Press.

Wingood, G. M., DiClemente, R. J., Mikhail, I., Lang, D. L., McCree, D. H., Davies, S. L., & Saag, M. (2004). A randomized controlled trial to reduce HIV transmission risk behaviors and sexually transmitted diseases among women living with HIV: The WiLLOW Program. *Journal of Acquired Immune Deficiency Syndromes, 37*, S58–S67.

Wingood, G. M., & DiClemente, R. J. (2006). Enhancing adoption of evidence-based HIV interventions: Promotion of a suite of HIV prevention interventions for African American women. *AIDS Education and Prevention, 18*, 161–170.

Chapter 5
Tobacco Blinders: How Tobacco Control Remained Generic for Far Too Long

Lorraine Greaves and Natalie Hemsing

Tobacco: Global Public Health Issues

The tobacco industry is a multinational oligopoly with a global reach. It is adaptive, moving from market to market, and continuously exploring new products, such as e-cigarettes[1] and heat-not-burn[2] tobacco systems (Elias & Ling, 2018; Huang et al., 2019). As a result, there is a continuing constellation of health and economic issues attributed to tobacco that represents the most serious global public health problem and the *leading cause of preventable death* in the world. Globally, more men than women smoke, but increasing smoking among girls and young women may change this pattern. In several countries such as France, Italy, Sweden, Argentina, and Chile, smoking among adolescent girls now exceeds that of adolescent boys (Drope et al., 2018).

Tobacco use directly kills over 7.1 M people per year, mostly through smoking-related cardiovascular diseases and cancers. There are nearly 900,000 deaths per year attributed to exposure to secondhand smoke, over half of whom are women who are exposed to men's smoking (Drope et al., 2018). In addition, there are countless environmental and economic costs linked to tobacco growing, processing, and manufacturing that often take resources such as arable land away from food production or degrade environments due to deforestation.

While many in higher-income countries, such as Canada and the United States, believe the tobacco issue has been solved, nothing could be further from the truth.

---

[1] A range of nicotine delivery systems that depend on vaporizing nicotine liquids, without smoking tobacco, that are touted as safer than smoking tobacco

[2] Tobacco-based products that heat, but do not combust, tobacco, touted as safer than combustible cigarettes.

L. Greaves (✉) · N. Hemsing
Centre of Excellence for Women's Health, Vancouver, BC, Canada
e-mail: lgreaves@cw.bc.ca; nhemsing@cw.bc.ca

© Springer Nature Switzerland AG 2021
J. Gahagan, M. K. Bryson (eds.), *Sex- and Gender-Based Analysis in Public Health*, https://doi.org/10.1007/978-3-030-71929-6_5

Even public health advocates sometimes need reminding that tobacco use is the leading preventable cause of death in the world. This chapter describes the failure of public health to include a sex-, gender-, and diversity-based analysis in tobacco control. Diversity analyses track, articulate, and describe differential patterns among populations and subpopulations, in order to highlight groups more or less vulnerable to tobacco use and signal areas for specific action. They also foster a critique of generic responses that mask specific and sometimes, ongoing vulnerabilities. Specifically, smoking and its impacts were assumed, wrongly, to be male phenomena, based on early adopters in high-income countries. This failure to apply a diversity analyses of data, and fashion responses accordingly, has undoubtedly led to unnecessary mortality and morbidity.

But the astonishing fact is that we have yet to see the global toll of tobacco use. While 100 million people died from tobacco use in the twentieth century, *one billion* people will die from tobacco use in the twenty-first century (Drope et al., 2018). Simply put, tobacco use kills 1 in 2 of its users (World Health Organization, 2011). By 2030, the number of tobacco-related deaths will increase from the current 7 million to 8 million each year (World Health Organization, 2011). And reflecting the industry shift from higher-income countries to lower-income countries, by 2030 80% of those deaths will be in low- and middle-income countries. It is the responsibility of the public health community to not only monitor such shifts and practices but to lead in their resolutions and treatment. Unfortunately, public health has typically focused on micro challenges, such as influencing individual behavioural changes such as tobacco cessation, as opposed to addressing the social, political, and economic structural factors creating and maintaining tobacco use trends and patterns.

The global public health community has been activated, however. The impact of tobacco use is so serious and severe, that tobacco use and control are the subject of the *only* international public health treaty in the world: the Framework Convention on Tobacco Control (WHO-FCTC) (World Health Organization, 2003). This treaty was passed into force in 2002 and has 168 country signatories. Its Conference of the Parties (COP) meetings happen regularly to refine data collection and regulation to meet the legal obligations inherent in the FCTC.

The Uneven Impacts of Tobacco

The impact of tobacco use has not been, and is still not, evenly felt across all populations or subpopulations. For example, Black American men smoke more than White American men (Kong et al., 2018), low-income young pregnant women smoke more than higher-income and older women (Greaves et al., 2019), and people with mental health diagnoses smoke at far higher rates than the general population (Chaiton & Callard, 2019). But historically the patterns were similar, with the uptake of tobacco use first occurred among men, and among the upper social classes, with women and lower socioeconomic groups following later. The uptake of commercially produced cigarettes first occurred around 1890 in the most developed countries, ultimately to be followed by less developed countries. This pattern reflected the impact of cultural diffusion. In many parts of the world, there are still rising smoking rates, with male smokers outnumbering female smokers, in some cases, by wide margins. Chinese smoking rates are an example, where 68% of men smoke versus 2% of women (World Health Organization, 2019).

Within social and geographic locations, there have been further differences among subpopulations. For example, Indigenous people in North America, while long using tobacco in traditional ways, came later to commercial cigarettes compared to non-Indigenous populations. The rates of smoking cigarettes among Indigenous groups in Canada, and around the world, are now a serious public health issue, with some indication that Canadian Indigenous groups experience some of the highest smoking rates in the world (Jetty, 2017; Waa et al., 2019).

Lowered uptake and quit rates have followed the same patterns with early adopters quitting first and more developed countries taking public health and regulatory action first. That means that men's rates peaked before women's and higher SES populations quit before lower SES populations (Thun et al., 2012). These trends have contributed to ongoing health inequities and, as we will see, gender and ethnic/racial inequities as well. Recognizing these distinct patterns and nuances has not been part of the typical public health response to tobacco use. In the main, the response has been generic: devoid of sex, gender, and diversity considerations. Furthermore, intersectional analyses of tobacco use are rare (Bottorff et al., 2014), where multiple factors affecting tobacco use are analysed simultaneously via sampling and analyses of large data sets. Rather, this chapter describes the dominant generic approach, the opportunities missed, and some remedies.

How Did Tobacco Use Spread?

Tobacco use first emerged as a public health issue in the early sixteenth century in Europe when spitting, chewing, and smoking tobacco in pipes emerged as modern behaviours among men in the higher socioeconomic classes. While rates of tobacco use among women in Europe were lower, women were also using these traditional tobacco products such as pipes, cigars, and hand-rolled cigarettes (Cook, 1997; Graham, 1996). These tobacco products used dark tobacco that was cured either by air, fire, or sun (Cook, 1997). Even today, In India, traditional tobacco products such as smokeless tobacco and bidis still constitute the predominant problematic forms of tobacco use for women (Mishra et al., 2015).

Throughout the nineteenth century, tobacco use became an increasingly gendered activity (Graham, 1996). But class and other social characteristics played a role in this diffusion. In Cook's analysis of gender and tobacco use in the archaeological record, they argue that in the context of smoking among late Victorian women in Britain and the United States, women cannot be seen as a homogenous group, but rather "divided by class and ethnic affiliations" (Cook, 1997). Clearly, there was such a divide that affected women's smoking behaviours. For example, in the 1850s upper- and middle-class women in both Britain and America were discouraged from smoking *in public*; yet working-class women smoked, and some ethnic subgroups such as Irish American and African American women are often depicted smoking short clay pipes (Cook, 1997). In California, Hispanic women often smoked cigars, and "young ladies' cigars" were marketed to women, sold with names such as "sweet lips" and "pansy blossoms" (Cook, 1997).

But things slowly changed for women. By the late nineteenth century, there is very low recorded tobacco use among women (Graham, 1996). During the 1890s, Cook claims that some middle-class women in Europe, in a break with Victorian tradition, began to smoke publicly, a practice which was often viewed with scorn by visitors from North America (Cook, 1997). A decade later, there is evidence of young, middle-, and upper-class women in the northeastern United States beginning to smoke during the summer and at dinner parties, following trends from Europe (Cook, 1997). However, smoking in public among women remained controversial; in 1908, in New York "Sullivan's Law" was introduced making it illegal for women to smoke in public places, albeit this was discontinued only 2 weeks later due to public opposition (Cook, 1997).

In short, smoking was socially constructed as a gendered activity confined to places predominantly inhabited by men, such as in cars and bars; therefore, it was a behaviour often seen by conservative politicians and social groups as something women should be protected from (Cook, 1997). Women who did smoke in public were perceived as being sexually available to men (Cook, 1997). White and colleagues argue that the stigma associated with women's smoking in the nineteenth century, which labelled men as "tobacco connoisseurs" and that of women as lacking self-control or capacity to "choose a quality tobacco," reflected the "gendered culture of consumption" in which masculinity is equated with rationality and femininity with irrationality (White et al., 2012). These were but a few of the gendered cultural meanings ascribed to tobacco use.

Tobacco use increased rapidly, primarily among men, during the twentieth century, as manufactured cigarettes using blond (flue-cured) tobaccos were introduced and advertising efforts increased (Graham, 1996). Commercial cigarettes had been invented in the late eighteenth century and quickly facilitated the rapid spread of smoking. However, cigarette smoking was still widely viewed as a vile habit for both women and men, particularly in the United States and Canada, where women's groups were instrumental in spearheading anti-tobacco movements (Amos & Haglund, 2000; Brandt, 1996). White and colleagues describe how in the late nineteenth century, cigarettes shifted to being perceived as "manly" due to advertising and promotional efforts, that featured athletes and beautiful women to appeal to men (White et al., 2012). Spurred by these advertising efforts, the manufactured cigarette became the popular delivery system for tobacco and nicotine. The manufacturing of cigarettes signalled the advent of big business and industry involvement in promoting smoking, and the powerful tobacco industry was born. The history of marketing and promotion of cigarettes involved widespread endorsements by famous or authoritative people and, notably, by doctors.

Smoking among women remained stigmatized until the 1920s and 1930s when rates began to increase (Brandt, 1996). This reflected the post-World War I efforts of the women's liberation movement and shifting gender roles, a time in which, as noted by Cook, the "traditional notions of the women's sphere" were increasingly being challenged (Cook, 1997). Brandt explains that, in the 1920s: "for men, the cigarette evoked images of power, authority, and independence; for women, it represented rebellious independence, glamour, seduction, and sexual allure and acted as a flexible symbol for both feminists and flappers" (Brandt, 1996 p.64). Edward Bernays, the nephew of Sigmund Freud, was instrumental in capitalizing on shifting gendered conventions by promoting smoking among women in public. In 1929, hired by George Washington Hill, the president of American Tobacco, Bernays promoted Lucky Strike cigarettes in the New York City Easter Day Parade; Bernays hired debutantes to march, smoking their "torches of freedom" to symbolize the suffragists' demands for women's rights (Amos & Haglund, 2000; Brandt, 1996). As Greaves (1996) points out the cultural meaning of smoking for women was manipulated by advertising through the early decades of the twentieth century:

> ...women's smoking as it relates to gender relations has moved from a symbol of being *bought* by men (prostitute), to being *like* men (lesbian/mannish/androgynous), to being *able to attract* men (glamourous/ heterosexual). (p. 21–22)

Smoking in public increased among women throughout the 1950s, and advertisers continued to equate smoking with women's liberation and freedom; Virginia Slims campaign evoked this in their late 1960s' campaign "You've come a long way baby!" (Amos & Haglund, 2000; Brandt, 1996). Virginia Slims was also the first to exploit race in marketing cigarettes to women, using the slogan "Find Your Voice," featuring racialized women in the pictorials.

The quantity of cigarettes consumed increased greatly during the early twentieth century, with men dominating the vast majority of consumption (White et al., 2012). By post World War II, the smoking rates among men were very high in Europe; for example, 75–90% of men reported smoking in Northern Europe (Graham, 1996). In Canada and the United States, similar rates were recorded with approximately three quarters of men and nearly half of women smoking during World War II (Ferrence, 1988).

Graham argues that smoking trends broadly align with the "diffusion of innovations" (Rogers & Shoemaker, 1971), in which new ideas or practices tend to first be initiated by relatively socially advantaged individuals and then spreading later to those of lower social advantage (Graham, 1996). This is reflected in smoking trends. In North America and Europe, smoking rates among men increased over the first half of the twentieth century and then began to decline between the 1960s and 1980s (Hunt et al., 2004). In contrast, women's smoking rates began to increase substantially during and following World War II and did not begin to decrease until about 10 years following the decrease observed among men (Hunt et al., 2004). For example, in the United States, the prevalence of ever smoking was highest among men in 1965 (71.7%) and among women in 1985 (46.2%) (Satcher et al., 2002).

Diffusion theory accounts for the spread from high-income countries to low-income countries in the last 20 years. Smoking rates have decreased steadily over time among women and men in Canada, the United States, and Europe while rising in lower-income countries. For example, in 2017, the overall smoking rate in Canada was 15.1%; and the 2019 report on trends in tobacco use in Canada note that "historically large sex differences in smoking prevalence have narrowed over time to within a few percentage points, although smoking has remained more prevalent among males" (Reid et al., 2019). Yet, declines in smoking are not uniform. Specifically, the decline in smoking among socially disadvantaged women and men has been less pronounced (Graham, 2012; Hunt et al., 2004). For example, in Canada, Indigenous women living on a low income, who have experienced violence and trauma and who use alcohol and other substances, report smoking at rates 2–5 times greater than the overall national rate (Hemsing et al., 2015). In low-income countries, smoking prevalence among women and girls has not yet peaked, having remained relatively low (Drope et al., 2018). However, these patterns may change as women in low- and middle-income countries are increasingly targeted by tobacco industry marketing efforts (Gilmore et al., 2015; Greaves et al., 2006).

Historical Responses of Public Health

King James was among the first to condemn smoking and issue limits to protect public health like confining smoking to specific locations such as tobacco houses (King James I of Great Britain, 1604). But 400 years later, the public health issues connected to tobacco use are widespread and rampant including involuntary exposure to others' smoke, access to tobacco products, new tobacco products and nicotine delivery systems, fires, littering, pollution, loss of food growing land to tobacco cultivation, environmental degradation, the erosion of tree habitats, exploitation of child, and women's labour in tobacco growing. The problem of tobacco use grew gradually but reached a key point of recognition mid-twentieth century when the signs of its incredible health impact were first signalled.

Beginning in the 1960s, the links between smoking and lung cancer increased in public awareness, and smoking rates began to decline (Graham, 2012). At that stage, most smokers were men, in higher-income countries, and predictably, most smokers dying from tobacco-related diseases were men in these same settings. Public health efforts focused largely on the risks for the smoker and were primarily aimed at men until the late 1970s. At this time, health promotion efforts in higher-income countries began to focus on the risk to others, particularly the risks to the fetus and children of pregnant women who smoked (Berridge & Loughlin, 2005).

Ironically, while women and girls were ignored in most public health campaigns prior to the 1970s and 1980s, they have never been ignored by the tobacco industry. Indeed, quite the opposite treatment was, and continues to be, applied to women, as marketers and producers tried, and succeeded, in luring women and girls to smoke manufactured cigarettes in many regions of the globe. Women were included in advertisements encouraging women to take up smoking to lose weight, become (hetero)sexually attractive, acquire glamour, and experience relaxation, independence, and other benefits. These messages and images were extremely effective in recruiting women to smoke. Even sex-specific differences have been catered for by the tobacco industry as they developed female-specific products, such as low-nicotine, light, slim cigarettes in order to appeal to girls and women and to suit their physiological responses to nicotine (Silverstein et al., 1980). Indeed, biology matters as female adolescents transition to nicotine dependence faster than male adolescents, likely due to sex hormones interacting with dopamine receptors (Sylvestre et al., 2018). These differences represent missed opportunities for sex-specific prevention in public health.

How Sex and Gender Matter in Tobacco

Identifying such sex and gender issues in research, prevention, and treatment for tobacco was entirely missing until the 1990s. This was due to tobacco-related illnesses (such as cardiovascular disease and lung cancer) being perceived by medicine as "male" diseases in the mid-twentieth century: an artefact of the distribution of smoking. More broadly there was scientific sexism that created resistance to understanding women's health (Greaves, 2018b); indifference on the part of the women's health movement to advocating on women's tobacco use (Greaves, 2018a); and a lack of engagement with the social factors affecting tobacco use, prevention, and treatment (Greaves, 2007). While this scientific sexism has been partially exposed with the rise of sex and gender science in some developed countries such as Canada, the United States, and the United Kingdom, there is a very long way to go in bringing the gender preamble of the WHO-FCTC to life.

Sex refers to the biological characteristics and physiological processes associated with male and female bodies, and in the context of tobacco includes the biological responses to tobacco use and treatments. For example, females who smoke cigarettes are more vulnerable to chronic obstructive pulmonary disease (COPD) with lower levels of cigarette exposure; this is due in part to smaller lungs, airways, and the influence of sex hormones (Aryal et al., 2014; Hemsing & Greaves, 2008). There is evidence that ovarian hormones also impact responses to nicotine use, metabolism, and withdrawal. Nicotine withdrawal is affected by menstrual patterns; when quitting smoking, women tend to report greater withdrawal symptoms in the luteal phase (Carpenter et al., 2006). Sex hormones impact CYP2A6 activity which is the enzyme activity involved in nicotine metabolism; and nicotine metabolism is faster in females compared to males, particularly among women taking birth control containing oestrogen and during pregnancy (Benowitz, 2008).

In contrast, males metabolize nicotine more slowly than females and are more likely to smoke for the reinforcing effects of nicotine (Verplaetse et al., 2015). Sex-related factors also impact tobacco treatment responses. Systematic reviews reveal poorer cessation outcomes for women compared to men with pharmacological supports, such as nicotine replacement therapy (NRT), regardless of whether or not combined with counselling (Perkins & Scott, 2008), and bupropion (Smith, Weinberger, et al., 2017a). In contrast, women treated with varenicline have demonstrated similar or better outcomes compared to men (Glatard et al., 2017; McKee et al., 2016; Smith, Zhang, et al., 2017b).

Gender-related factors include roles, norms, identities, and rules associated with men, women, boys, girls, and transgender individuals. Gender-related factors impact smoking initiation, patterns of tobacco use, the meanings ascribed to smoking, capacity to control secondhand smoke (SHS) exposure, and responses to tobacco policies and interventions. For example, men tend to be more often exposed to SHS at work and women more often in the home (Greaves & Hemsing, 2009b). Girls and women often smoke as a means to control negative moods and emotions (Greaves, 2015). And as described previously, the tobacco industry has linked smoking with empowerment and sexual attractiveness for women and with strength and masculinity for men (Amos et al., 2012). There is virtually no research on smoking among transgender people based on representative samples, but one recent US study indicates that transgender individuals smoke at high rates (Buchting et al., 2017). Both natal sex and assumed gender play a part in interpreting the influences of tobacco marketing as well as responses to public health initiatives.

Historically gendered patterns in tobacco use are reflected in mortality rates; while smoking-related mortality has been stable among men since the 1980s, there is some evidence that the risk of death from smoking has increased among women (Zhang et al., 2015). With the narrowing gender gap in smoking, it is expected that gender differences in smoking-related mortality will decrease over time (Denney et al., 2010; Rostron & Wilmoth, 2011). Gender norms and roles also impact the experience of smoking-related stigma. For example, pregnant women who smoke report experiencing significant stigma and are less likely to disclose their smoking to a healthcare provider or seek support (Hemsing et al., 2012). Similarly, new fathers also experience smoking-related stigma, and many new fathers concentrate their smoking in vehicles or at worksites as a result to avoid the perceived conflict with their role as protectors and providers (Greaves et al., 2010).

Contemporary Responses by Public Health

Sadly, the public health response remained generic and sex and gender blind. It did not mimic these sex- and gender-specific elements in designing either prevention, health promotion, or gender-specific treatments. It did not examine the gendered impact of tobacco policy on men and women or girls and boys, nor did tobacco control research, either in investigating the effects of tobacco use on males and females or, in the responses of men and women to various initiatives and campaigns (Amos et al., 2012).

Similarly, a wide range of differences and their interactive effects in subpopulations are glossed over by reliance on population-based data collection and, subsequently, by public health practitioners. The gendered and inequitable impact of tobacco use has consistently been obscured by relying on population-based data (Greaves, 2007; Greaves & Hemsing, 2009a). These overarching data show a general decline in tobacco use, causing many public health advocates to relax and contributing the feeling that the tobacco issue is solved.

There have been two exceptions to this. They both focus, not surprisingly on women, reflecting ongoing sexism and objectification. The first one concerns pregnancy. A sex-specific preoccupation of public health and medicine with pregnancy and smoking dominated the "women's smoking" issue for decades. Indeed, until 1990, there was little research and little intervention on women's and girls' smoking other than pregnancy quit campaigns that were consistently fetus centric. "Quit smoking during pregnancy for the sake of the fetus", was the public health rallying cry. This shaming approach had nothing to do with women's health or in understanding that women are more than vessels for reproduction. It had nothing to do with understanding the social determinants of health that affect women's tobacco use during pregnancy or the post pregnancy 90% relapse rate when women did quit. It took a concerted effort by feminist health advocates and researchers to begin to replace this sexist approach with a fundamentally different, women-centred approach (Greaves et al., 2011).

The other public health approach that has had a long reach is tying women's smoking to facial wrinkles and other signs of aging. "Faggash Lil" was featured in a British commercial and represented as unappealing (Jacobson, 1986). An early American Cancer Society poster featuring a very wrinkled and haggard-looking woman with stained fingers and the caption "Smoking is very Glamorous" has lingered. These messages have been ageist, sexist, and superficial and have reinforced negative gender stereotypes of how women might be preoccupied with beauty as a key motivator and how public health should actively exploit that as opposed to transform it.

Furthermore, these approaches don't seem to work. Programmes and .approaches such as these can reinforce dominant gender norms. For example, tobacco prevention programmes have been implemented and evaluated that use a computer model to predict facial appearance if smoking is continued (Brinker et al., 2017; Grogan et al., 2011). While pilot studies of these programmes have found these to be effective among girls and young women, they also reinforce societal norms that prioritize youth and beauty among women. For example, Grogan and colleagues found that while young women reported a high motivation to quit smoking after viewing how they would appear if they continue to smoke, the intervention also "produced a fear and anxiety reaction," reflective of the "Western societal context where women are expected to look youthful and where looking young and being perceived as attractive are culturally enmeshed" (Grogan et al., 2011).

Global Responses by Public Health

There has been lip service on the global level to issues of gender and Indigenous issues. The WHO-FCTC treaty covers numerous measures and issues in tobacco control, including price and tax measures to reduce the demand for tobacco and non-price measures to reduce the demand for tobacco, such as protection from exposure to tobacco smoke; regulation of the contents of tobacco products and product disclosures; packaging and labelling of tobacco products; education, communication, training, and public awareness; tobacco advertising, promotion, and sponsorship; as well as numerous demand reduction measures concerning tobacco dependence and cessation (World Health Organization, 2003).

This public health intervention on tobacco was the culmination of the work and dedication of a large number of players, both inside and outside governments, working together across national borders in order to define and implement a broad response to the global health threats posed by tobacco use. It has served to cohere and cement the global tobacco control movement and to focus on setting standards for all countries in reducing the impact of tobacco on public health. It is a significant achievement for public health. Women's health activists introduced the concept of gender to the deliberations designing the treaty and managed to make some differences to the wording of this treaty in its initial formulation.

One of the key preambles to the WHO-FCTC states that "*Alarmed* by the increase in smoking and other forms of tobacco consumption by women and young girls worldwide and keeping in mind the need for full participation of women at all levels of policy-making and implementation and the need for gender-specific tobacco control strategies" (World Health Organization, 2003). There is a similar preamble on Indigenous health, where the FCTC text states that the signatories are: "*Deeply concerned* about the high levels of smoking and other forms of tobacco consumption by indigenous peoples".

These preambles are significant, reflecting real concerns about the social justice and gendered impact of tobacco use in the world and the need for a sensitive and gendered response. While this is highly reflective of evidence and trends, this concern with gender has not always permeated the work of either the FCTC or the tobacco control movement more generally (Amos et al., 2012). Amos et al. indicate that in all spheres, the lack of attention to gender and its influence on tobacco use is significant, particularly with respect to women's tobacco use. They found that tobacco control has been largely gender-blind and that the animation of the FCTC on gender and women's tobacco use in particular has been deficient.

Global female tobacco use is increasingly complex, with gaps between boys and girls closing in some regions, escalating women's use in some regions, and disadvantage driving persisting smoking rates in other regions (Chaiton & Callard, 2019; Landstedt & San Sebastian, 2018; Pampel et al., 2017). All of these diverse trends could be better tackled if a consistent sex and gender analysis was applied to all matters of the FCTC. But, such analyses and approaches to tobacco control are uncommon, especially in low-income and middle-income countries.

Men's tobacco use can also benefit from much needed gender analyses, in order to ascertain reasons for smoking, quitting, and the impacts of policy and programming. However, men's tobacco use has typically been used as the norm and indeed the impetus for the birth of the tobacco control movement, and the lagging attention to women's use has in part been because women's trends in tobacco use were delayed. In short, the lack of integration of sex and gender considerations in research, policy, and programmes affects women, men, and gender-diverse people.

What Could Transform a Public Health Response to Gender and Tobacco?

Feminist thinkers have been, and still are, key to shifting the gaze of tobacco control to gender and equity. For 30 years feminist thinkers have suggested that dissecting the population of smokers and taking a clear sex- and gender-based analysis to tobacco use are essential. While widely dismissed as fringe thinkers at first, the tobacco control movement is slowly showing signs of embracing not only gender equity but social justice, especially with the rise of tobacco use in low-income countries.

It has been essential, however, to remove or redirect the preoccupation of clinicians and researchers away from pregnancy and reproduction and to introduce a social determinants of health perspective with a concern for women's health in its own right. It has been essential to introduce sex and gender science to tobacco. For example, introducing sex as a variable to understand tolerance to nicotine has led to critiques of standard tests of dependence such as the Fagerstrom test, showing that for women, this standard clinical test of the level of dependence was less sensitive than it was for men (Richardson et al., 2007). It allowed us to see that variable rates of consumption (number of cigarettes per day) were sex-sensitive, not just gender-sensitive. It opened up the door to seeing how responses to treatment such as cessation aids needed to be analysed by sex, as biological factors affect responses to all drugs.

Introducing gender as a variable has allowed us to understand access to tobacco (Kaestle, 2009), meanings attributed to smoking (Greaves, 2015), style and ritual (Greaves, 1996), and responses to policy, advertising, and marketing (Amos & Haglund, 2000; Greaves & Hemsing, 2009a; Hemsing et al., 2012). This new approach has led to tailoring messages, prevention and cessation campaigns, treatment, and the development of a more specific and personalized healthcare response. Acknowledging gender has also led to a reframing of how attention to pregnancy and reproduction can include men and boys (Bottorff et al., 2015; Bottorff et al., 2019; Greaves et al., 2010; Greaves et al., 2011). In short, the introduction of sex, gender, and related concepts into tobacco control has sharpened the global response to tobacco. It has led to a more equitable approach in tobacco control and a rebuttal to a solely population-based effectiveness ethos. It has undermined the "one size fits all" ethos and allowed for tailoring of responses to become more mainstream.

Gender-Transformative Approaches Are Required

Focusing on the outcomes of sex- and gender-based analysis is critically important to rectifying discrepancies in human health. Gender-transformative health promotion represents a raising of the bar in understanding sex and gender in health and identifying gender equity as a goal. Gender-transformative approaches to tobacco actively examine, question, and challenge stereotypical gender norms and imbalances of power as a means of reducing tobacco use *along with* increasing gender equity. Gender-transformative approaches would move public health from being gender-blind or neutral to more effective gender-sensitive, specific, or, better, transformative.

Tobacco control has been challenged to not only integrate sex- and gender-based analysis but, in light of the significant gender and equity issues connected to tobacco use, to become gender-transformative in its approach (Greaves, 2014). More specifically, the opportunities within the WHO-FCTC for gender-transformative work have been highlighted (Greaves & Tungohan, 2007). While examples of the application of gender-transformative approaches to tobacco treatment practices are still few, qualitative research with Canadian women accessing substance use treatment (Minian et al., 2016) and US women veterans (Katzburg et al., 2009) who smoke has revealed similar needs for women-centred smoking cessation interventions, including components that empower women or improve their access to treatment such as programming created by and for women; choice and individualized treatment; psychosocial supports and free pharmacotherapy; women-specific education; and childcare support.

Similarly, based on research exploring the needs of women who smoke, researchers from the Centre of Excellence for Women's Health (CEWH) developed guidance for providers for engaging in brief interventions with women who smoke (Urquhart et al., 2012). A women-centred approach builds on the strengths of women, is harm reduction-oriented, trauma-informed, and prioritizes safety and social justice issues (Urquhart et al., 2012). More recently, similar principles have been adapted for working with young and socially disadvantaged women during pregnancy (Greaves et al., 2019). Smoking cessation interventions that engage women in the programme development and that emphasize social support have reported positive improvements for low-income women who smoke (Stewart et al., 2010) and African American women (Andrews et al., 2007).

Similar calls have been made for tailored smoking cessation interventions for men (Okoli et al., 2011). Men-centred smoking cessation websites have been developed and evaluated with men by the Families Controlling and Eliminating Tobacco (FACET) research programme (Bottorff et al., 2015; Bottorff et al., 2018; Bottorff et al., 2016a). These online resources have been tailored to address men's smoking-related needs by offering men choices in smoking cessation resources; linking positive identities such as being strong and healthy with being smoke-free; and offering social support via an interactive discussion forum and a buddy support system. Evaluations with men who used the online resources demonstrated that, at 6-month follow-up, 24% of men had quit smoking and 40% had reduced their smoking (Bottorff et al., 2016b). An online smoking cessation resource has also been developed specifically for new fathers, *Dads in Gear* (Bottorff et al., 2015), which offers gender-specific parenting resources for men, makes links between masculine identities and fathering, and encourages men to be a healthy role model as a father by quitting smoking.

What Comes Next?

In an era of tobacco industry innovation in e-cigarettes and young people using such products to consume and become dependent on nicotine, the world is facing a new upsurge in smoking and vaping (Drope et al., 2018). Devious marketing has offered e-cigarettes as harm reduction approaches to quitting smoking traditional cigarettes but, not surprisingly, has swept up brand new smokers into nicotine dependence. There is emerging evidence that some of the youth using e-cigarettes are indeed becoming dependent on nicotine and moving on to the uptake of traditional cigarette smoking (Hammond et al., 2017). These products are being marketed with gendered overtones and campaigns and with product marketing and colours and flavours that are destined to attract young girls and boys (Kong et al., 2017).

The tobacco industry has been a consistently good example of using a sex- and gender-based analysis in order to further its interests. The industry has even verged into gender-transformative territory in launching campaigns evoking themes of liberation for women, "You've Come a Long Way Baby" (Phillip Morris International, 1968), and empowerment for racialized women "Find Your Voice" (Phillip Morris international, 2000). Public health has failed at this. As a result, public health has consistently lagged behind the industry and been on its heel, reacting, not designing proactive interventions. This is a long-term problem that is repeating itself. The introduction of e-cigarettes, for example, was marketed as a harm reduction tool for smokers to quit. Leading up to this, harm reduction has been bitterly contested and resisted in tobacco control as not a worthy goal, given that *any* amount of tobacco use is unsafe. Nicotine replacement therapies were the closest that tobacco control had come to harm reduction, and they fail to mimic the behavioural aspects of smoking traditional cigarettes. The vacuum created by this was filled by the e-cigarette trend and welcomed by addicted smokers.

Facing this new upsurge in nicotine dependence may remove some of the harms of traditional tobacco but is introducing new harms in the form of vaping-related illnesses, primarily lung illnesses (Hopkins Tanne, 2019). The opportunity is ripe for health research and public health to apply a sex and gender lens to these new phenomena, but will it happen? A recent review indicated almost a complete lack of sex- and gender-based vaping research, offering little on which to base new campaigns (unpublished).

The imposition of sex- and gender-based analysis, a social justice and social determinants framework, and a value-based, principle-driven approach is required.

This requires some adjustments. Not only will public health have to re-embrace tobacco control, but it also will have to do so with a much more sophisticated and radical edge. New conceptualizations such as trauma-informed practices, social equity, gender-transformative, and harm reduction approaches will need to be overtly integrated into responding to tobacco (and e-cigarettes) going forward. Current crises in the emergence of new nicotine delivery products are exacerbating these issues, as the tobacco industry tries to reinvent itself on the backs of human health.

Are we destined to repeat the mistakes of the past? Will we continue to be gender- and sex-blind? Will we continue to privilege population-based statistics over subgroup trends? Will we resist tailoring our responses to gendered patterns of tobacco use and e-cigarette use with subpopulations and by global regions? Will we increase our use of "within-group" analyses in research to identify the many intersecting factors affecting tobacco use? Will we continue to evade our WHO-FCTC pledge to centre gender and Indigenous issues in our planning, research, messaging, and policy-making? Will we continue to avoid taking responsibility for improving gender equity as we go about responding to cigarettes and their new cousins, e-cigarettes? Will we balk at social justice approaches to analysing global trends, and will we ignore the impact of tobacco marketing on racialized populations, marginal groups, and low-income people and countries? When will public health respond to tobacco in accordance with the size and gravity of the issue and its clear sex, gender, and equity concerns?

References

Amos, A., Greaves, L., Nichter, M., & Bloch, M. (2012). Women and tobacco: A call for including gender in tobacco control research, policy and practice. *Tobacco Control, 21*(2), 236–243.

Amos, A., & Haglund, M. (2000). From social taboo to "torch of freedom": The marketing of cigarettes to women. *Tobacco Control, 9*(1), 3–8. https://doi.org/10.1136/tc.9.1.3

Andrews, J. O., Felton, G., Ellen Wewers, M., Waller, J., & Tingen, M. (2007). The effect of a multi-component smoking cessation intervention in African American women residing in public housing. *Research in Nursing & Health, 30*(1), 45–60.

Aryal, S., Diaz-Guzman, E., & Mannino, D. M. (2014). Influence of sex on chronic obstructive pulmonary disease risk and treatment outcomes. *International Journal of Chronic Obstructive Pulmonary Disease, 9*(1), 1145–1154.

Benowitz, N. (2008). Clinical pharmacology of nicotine: Implications for understanding, preventing, and treating tobacco addiction. *Clinical Pharmacology & Therapeutics, 83*(4), 531–541.

Berridge, V., & Loughlin, K. (2005). Smoking and the new health education in Britain 1950s–1970s. *American Journal of Public Health, 95*(6), 956–964.

Bottorff, J. L., Oliffe, J. L., Sarbit, G., Caperchione, C. M., Currie, L. M., Schmid, J., et al. (2016a). Evaluation of QuitNow men: An online, men-centered smoking cessation intervention. *Journal of Medical Internet Research, 18*(4), 73–82. https://doi.org/10.2196/jmir.5076

Bottorff, J. L., Oliffe, J. L., Sarbit, G., Kelly, M. T., & Cloherty, A. (2015). Men's responses to online smoking cessation resources for new fathers: The influence of masculinities. *JMIR Research Protocols, 4*(2), e54. https://doi.org/10.2196/resprot.4079

Bottorff, J. L., Haines-Saah, R., Kelly, M. T., Oliffe, J. L., Torchalla, I., Poole, N., et al. (2014). Gender, smoking and tobacco reduction and cessation: A scoping review. *International Journal for Equity in Health, 13*(1), 114. https://doi.org/10.1186/s12939-014-0114-2

Bottorff, J. L., Oliffe, J. L., Sarbit, G., Sharp, P., Caperchione, C. M., Currie, L. M., et al. (2016b). Evaluation of QuitNow men: An online, men-centered smoking cessation intervention. *Journal of Medical Internet Research, 18*(4), e83. https://doi.org/10.2196/jmir.5076

Bottorff, J. L., Oliffe, J. L., Sarbit, G., Sharp, P., & Kelly, M. T. (2018). Smoke-free men: Competing and connecting to quit. *American Journal of Health Promotion, 32*(1), 135–142. https://doi.org/10.1177/0890117116671257

Bottorff, J. L., Sarbit, G., Oliffe, J. L., Caperchione, C. M., Wilson, D., & Huisken, A. (2019). Strategies for supporting smoking cessation among indigenous fathers: A qualitative participatory study. *American Journal of Men's Health, 13*(1), 1557988318806438.

Brandt, A. M. (1996). Recruiting women smokers: The engineering of consent. *Journal of the American Medical Women's Association,* (1–2), 51, 63–66.

Brinker, T. J., Owczarek, A. D., Seeger, W., Groneberg, D. A., Brieske, C. M., Jansen, P., et al. (2017). A medical student-delivered smoking prevention program, education against tobacco, for secondary schools in Germany: Randomized controlled trial. *Journal of Medical Internet Research, 19*(6), e199. https://doi.org/10.2196/jmir.7906

Buchting, F. O., Emory, K. T., Scout, Kim, Y., Fagan, P., Vera, L. E., et al. (2017). Transgender use of cigarettes, cigars, and e-cigarettes in a national study. *American Journal of Preventive Medicine, 53*(1), e1–e7. https://doi.org/10.1016/j.amepre.2016.11.022

Carpenter, M. J., Upadhyaya, H. P., LaRowe, S. D., Saladin, M. E., & Brady, K. T. (2006). Menstrual cycle phase effects on nicotine withdrawal and cigarette craving: A review. *Nicotine & Tobacco Research, 8*(5), 627–638.

Chaiton, M., & Callard, C. (2019). Mind the gap: Disparities in cigarette smoking in Canada. *Tobacco Use Insights, 12,* 1179173X19839058. https://doi.org/10.1177/1179173X19839058

Cook, L. J. (1997). "Promiscuous smoking": Interpreting gender and tobacco use in the archaeological record. *Northeast Historical Archaeology, 26*(1), 3.

Denney, J. T., Rogers, R. G., Hummer, R. A., & Pampel, F. C. (2010). Education inequality in mortality: The age and gender specific mediating effects of cigarette smoking. *Social Science Research, 39*(4), 662–673. https://doi.org/10.1016/j.ssresearch.2010.02.007

Drope, J., Schluger, N., Cahn, Z., Drope, J., Hamill, S., Islami, F., et al. (2018). *The tobacco atlas.* Atlanta: American Cancer Society and Vital Strategies.

Elias, J., & Ling, P. M. (2018). Invisible smoke: Third-party endorsement and the resurrection of heat-not-burn tobacco products. *Tobacco Control, 27*(Suppl 1), s96–s101. https://doi.org/10.1136/tobaccocontrol-2018-054433

Ferrence, R. G. (1988). *The diffusion of cigarette smoking: An exploratory analysis.* University of Western Ontario.

Gilmore, A. B., Fooks, G., Drope, J., Bialous, S. A., & Jackson, R. R. (2015). Exposing and addressing tobacco industry conduct in low-income and middle-income countries. *The Lancet, 385*(9972), 1029–1043.

Glatard, A., Dobrinas, M., Gholamrezaee, M., Lubomirov, R., Cornuz, J., Csajka, C., et al. (2017). Association of nicotine metabolism and sex with relapse following varenicline and nicotine replacement therapy. *Experimental & Clinical Psychopharmacology, 25*(5), 353–362. https://doi.org/10.1037/pha0000141

Graham, H. (1996). Smoking prevalence among women in the European Community 1950–1990. *Social Science & Medicine, 43*(2), 243–254. https://doi.org/10.1016/0277-9536(95)00369-X

Graham, H. (2012). Smoking, stigma and social class. *Journal of Social Policy, 41*(1), 83–99.

Greaves, L. (1996). *Smoke screen: Women's smoking and social control.* London: Scarlet Press.

Greaves, L. (2007). Gender, equity and tobacco control. *Health Sociology Review, 16*(2), 115–129.

Greaves, L. (2014). Can tobacco control be transformative? Reducing gender inequity and tobacco use among vulnerable populations. *International Journal of Environmental Research and Public Health, 11*(1), 792–803.

Greaves, L. (2015). The meanings of smoking to women and their implications for cessation. *International Journal of Environmental Research and Public Health, 12*(2), 1449–1465.

Greaves, L., & Hemsing, N. (2009a). Women and tobacco control policies: Social-structural and psychosocial contributions to vulnerability to tobacco use and exposure. *Drug and Alcohol Dependence, 104,* S121–S130.

Greaves, L., Jategaonkar, N., & Sanchez, S. (2006). *Turning a new leaf: Women, tobacco, and the future*. Vancouver, BC: British Columbia Centre of Excellence for Women's Health; International Network of Women Against Tobacco.

Greaves, L., Oliffe, J. L., Ponic, P., Kelly, M. T., & Bottorff, J. L. (2010). Unclean fathers, responsible men: Smoking, stigma and fatherhood. *Health Sociology Review, 19*(4), 522–533.

Greaves, L., Poole, N., & Hemsing, N. (2019). Tailored intervention for smoking reduction and cessation for young and socially disadvantaged women during pregnancy. *Journal of Obstetric, Gynecologic & Neonatal Nursing, 48*(1), 90–98.

Greaves, L., Poole, N., Okoli, C. T. C., Hemsing, N., Qu, A., Bialystok, L., et al. (2011). *Expecting to Quit: A best practices review of smoking cessation interventions for pregnant and postpartum girls and women*. Vancouver, BC: British Columbia Centre of Excellence for Women's Health and Health Canada.

Greaves, L., & Tungohan, E. (2007). Engendering tobacco control: Using an international public health treaty to reduce smoking and empower women. *Tobacco Control, 16*(3), 148–150. https://doi.org/10.1136/tc.2006.016337

Greaves, L. J., & Hemsing, N. J. (2009b). Sex, gender, and secondhand smoke policies: Implications for disadvantaged women. *American Journal of Preventive Medicine, 37*(2), S131–S137.

Greaves, L. (2018a). Sucking Back anger: Women and smoking. In L. Greaves (Ed.), *Personal and Political: Stories from the Women's Health Movement 1960–2010* (pp. 323–328). Second Story Press.

Greaves, L. (2018b). We Don't know what we Don't know: Advocating for women's health research. In L. Greaves (Ed.), *Personal and Political: Stories from the Women's Health Movement 1960–2010* (pp. 347–354). Second Story Press.

Grogan, S., Flett, K., Clark-Carter, D., Gough, B., Davey, R., Richardson, D., et al. (2011). Women smokers' experiences of an age-appearance anti-smoking intervention: A qualitative study. *British Journal of Health Psychology, 16*(4), 675–689. https://doi.org/10.1348/2044-8287.002006

Hammond, D., Reid, J. L., Cole, A. G., & Leatherdale, S. T. (2017). Electronic cigarette use and smoking initiation among youth: A longitudinal cohort study. *CMAJ, 189*(43), E1328–E1336.

Hemsing, N., Greaves, L., & Poole, N. (2015). Tobacco cessation interventions for underserved women. *Journal of Social Work Practice in the Addictions, 15*(3), 267–287. https://doi.org/10.1080/1533256X.2015.1054231

Hemsing, N., Greaves, L., Poole, N., & Bottorff, J. (2012). Reshuffling and relocating: The gendered and income-related differential effects of restricting smoking locations. *Journal of Environmental Research and Public Health, 2012*, 12. https://doi.org/10.1155/2012/907832

Hemsing, N., & Greaves, L. (2008). Article commentary: Women, environments and chronic disease: Shifting the gaze from individual level to structural factors. *Environmental Health Insights, 2*, EHI.S989. https://doi.org/10.4137/EHI.S989

Hopkins Tanne, J. (2019). Vaping: CDC investigates severe lung injuries. *BMJ, 366*, l5228. https://doi.org/10.1136/bmj.l5228

Huang, J., Duan, Z., Kwok, J., Binns, S., Vera, L. E., Kim, Y., et al. (2019). Vaping versus JUULing: How the extraordinary growth and marketing of JUUL transformed the US retail e-cigarette market. *Tobacco Control, 28*(2), 146–151. https://doi.org/10.1136/tobaccocontrol-2018-054382

Hunt, K., Hannah, M. K., & West, P. (2004). Contextualizing smoking: Masculinity, femininity and class differences in smoking in men and women from three generations in the west of Scotland. *Health Education Research, 19*(3), 239–249. https://doi.org/10.1093/her/cyg061

Jacobson, B. (1986). *Beating the lady killers: Women and smoking*. Pluto Press (UK).

Jetty, R. (2017). Tobacco use and misuse among indigenous children and youth in Canada. *Paediatrics & Child Health, 22*(7), 395–399.

Kaestle, C. E. (2009). How girls and boys get tobacco: Adults and other sources. *Journal of Adolescent Health, 45*(2), 208–210.

Katzburg, J. R., Yano, E. M., Washington, D. L., Farmer, M. M., Yee, E. F. T., Fu, S., et al. (2009). Combining Women's preferences and expert advice to design a tailored smoking cessation program (article). *Substance Use & Misuse, 44*(14), 2114–2127. https://doi.org/10.3109/10826080902858433

King James I of Great Britain. (1604). A Counterblaste to Tobacco. In *The Workes of the Most High and Mighty Prince, James* (pp. 214–222). London, UK.

Kong, G., Kuguru, K. E., & Krishnan-Sarin, S. (2017). Gender differences in US adolescent E-cigarette use. *Current Addiction Reports, 4*(4), 422–430.

Kong, A. Y., Golden, S. D., & Berger, M. T. (2018). An intersectional approach to the menthol cigarette problem: what's race (ism) got to do with it? *Critical Public Health*, 1–8.

McKee, S. A., Smith, P. H., Kaufman, M., Mazure, C. M., & Weinberger, A. H. (2016). Sex differences in Varenicline efficacy for smoking cessation: A meta-analysis. *Nicotine & Tobacco Research, 18*(5), 1002–1011. https://doi.org/10.1093/ntr/ntv207

Landstedt, E., & San Sebastian, M. (2018). Complex inequalities of gender and social class in daily smoking among Swedish men and women. *European Journal of Public Health, 28*(suppl_4). https://doi.org/10.1093/eurpub/cky214.048

Minian, N., Penner, J., Voci, S., & Selby, P. (2016). Woman focused smoking cessation programming: A qualitative study. *BMC Women's Health, 16*, 17. https://doi.org/10.1186/s12905-016-0298-2

Mishra, G. A., Kulkarni, S. V., Gupta, S. D., & Shastri, S. S. (2015). Smokeless tobacco use in urban Indian women: Prevalence and predictors. *Official Journal of Indian Society of Medical & Paediatric Oncology, 36*(3), 176.

Okoli, C. T. C., Torchalla, I., Oliffe, J. L., & Bottorff, J. L. (2011). Men's smoking cessation interventions: A brief review (review). *Journal of Men's Health, 8*(2), 100–108.

Pampel, F. C., Bricard, D., Khlat, M., & Legleye, S. (2017). Life course changes in smoking by gender and education: A cohort comparison across France and the United States. *Population Research and Policy Review, 36*(3), 309–330.

Perkins, K. A., & Scott, J. (2008). Sex differences in long-term smoking cessation rates due to nicotine patch. *Nicotine & Tobacco Research, 10*(7), 1245–1250. https://doi.org/10.1080/14622200802097506

Phillip Morris International. (1968). *You've come a long way, baby*. Leo Burnett Agency.

Phillip Morris International. (2000). *Virginia slims: Find your voice*.

Reid, J. L., Hammond, D., Tariq, U., Burkhalter, R., Rynard, V. L., & Douglas, O. (2019). *Tobacco use in Canada: Patterns and trends*. Waterloo, ON: Propel Centre for Population Health Impact, University of Waterloo.

Richardson, L., Greaves, L., Jategaonkar, N., Bell, K., Pederson, A., & Tungohan, E. (2007). Rethinking an assessment of nicotine dependence: A sex, gender and diversity analysis of the Fagerstrom test for nicotine dependence. *Journal of Smoking Cessation, 2*(2), 59–67.

Rogers, E. M., & Shoemaker, F. F. (1971). *Communication of innovations; A cross-cultural approach.*

Rostron, B. L., & Wilmoth, J. R. (2011). Estimating the effect of smoking on slowdowns in mortality declines in developed countries (article). *Demography, 48*(2), 461–479. https://doi.org/10.1007/s13524-011-0020-9

Satcher, D., Thompson, T., & Koplan, J. (2002). Women and smoking: A report of the surgeon general. *Nicotine & Tobacco Research, 4*(1), 7.

Silverstein, B., Feld, S., & Kozlowski, L. T. (1980). The availability of low-nicotine cigarettes as a cause of cigarette smoking among teenage females. *Journal of Health and Social Behavior*, 383–388.

Smith, P. H., Weinberger, A. H., Zhang, J., Emme, E., Mazure, C. M., & McKee, S. A. (2017a). Sex differences in smoking cessation pharmacotherapy comparative efficacy: A network meta-analysis. *Nicotine & Tobacco Research, 19*(3), 273–281. https://doi.org/10.1093/ntr/ntw144

Smith, P. H., Zhang, J., Weinberger, A. H., Mazure, C. M., & McKee, S. A. (2017b). Gender differences in the real-world effectiveness of smoking cessation medications: Findings from the 2010–2011 tobacco use supplement to the current population survey. *Drug & Alcohol Dependence, 178*, 485–491. https://doi.org/10.1016/j.drugalcdep.2017.05.046

Stewart, M. J., Kushner, K. E., Greaves, L., Letourneau, N., Spitzer, D., & Boscoe, M. (2010). Impacts of a support intervention for low-income women who smoke. *Social Science & Medicine, 71*(11), 1901–1909. https://doi.org/10.1016/j.socscimed.2010.08.023

Sylvestre, M.-P., Chagnon, M., Wellman, R. J., Dugas, E. N., & O'Loughlin, J. (2018). Sex differences in attaining cigarette smoking and nicotine dependence milestones among novice smokers. *American Journal of Epidemiology, 187*(8), 1670–1677. https://doi.org/10.1093/aje/kwy045

Thun, M., Peto, R., Boreham, J., & Lopez, A. D. (2012). Stages of the cigarette epidemic on entering its second century. *Tobacco Control, 21*(2), 96–101.

Urquhart, C., Jasiura, F., Poole, N., Nathoo, T., & Greaves, L. (2012). *Liberation!: Helping women quit smoking: A brief tobacco intervention guide.* British Columbia Centre of Excellence for Women's Health.

Verplaetse, T. L., Weinberger, A. H., Smith, P. H., Cosgrove, K. P., Mineur, Y. S., Picciotto, M. R., et al. (2015). Targeting the noradrenergic system for gender-sensitive medication development for tobacco dependence. *Nicotine & Tobacco Research, 17*(4), 486–495.

Waa, A., Robson, B., Gifford, H., Smylie, J., Reading, J., Henderson, J. A., et al. (2019). Foundation for a Smoke-Free World and healthy indigenous futures: An oxymoron? *Tobacco Control*, tobaccocontrol-2018-054792.

White, C., Oliffe, J. L., & Bottorff, J. L. (2012). Fatherhood, smoking, and secondhand smoke in North America: An historical analysis with a view to contemporary practice. *American Journal of Men's Health, 6*(2), 146–155. https://doi.org/10.1177/1557988311425852

World Health Organization. (2003). *WHO framework convention on tobacco control.* Geneva: World Health Organization.

World Health Organization. (2011). *WHO report on the global tobacco epidemic, 2011: The MPOWER package.* Geneva: World Health Organization.

World Health Organization. (2019). *Global Health Observatory data repository.* Geneva: World Health Organization.

Zhang, M. Z., An, Q., Yeh, F., Zhang, Y., Howard, B. V., Lee, E. T., et al. (2015). Smoking-attributable mortality in American Indians: Findings from the strong heart study. *European Journal of Epidemiology, 30*(7), 553–561. https://doi.org/10.1007/s10654-015-0031-8

Chapter 6
Beyond "Women's Cancers": Sex and Gender in Cancer Health and Care

Jacqueline Gahagan, Mary K. Bryson, and Fiona Warde

Introduction

The purpose of this chapter is to demonstrate why current public health approaches to 'women's cancers' must move beyond the longstanding sex-based female/male binary model in order to develop effective cancer screening messaging and cancer care program development. For example, the common conflation of 'sex' and 'gender' as equivalent terms is highly problematic given that these conceptualizations are used to inform cancer risk assessments and care delivery models. This results in approaches that are devoid of the underlying determinants of health that in fact contribute to cancer rates as well as survival rates. The focus of this chapter is on the Canadian cancer care context and will conclude with recommendations for gender-transformative cancer care globally in public health.

Context

Cancer is a significant and growing public health concern globally. According to the World Health Organization, approximately 30–50% of all cancers are deemed preventable (WHO, 2018). Further, the WHO states that key contributors to cancer

J. Gahagan (✉)
Faculty of Health, Dalhousie University, Halifax, NS, Canada
e-mail: jgahagan@dal.ca

M. K. Bryson
Department of Language and Literacy Education, Faculty of Education, University of British Columbia, Vancouver, BC, Canada

F. Warde
Department of Family Medicine, Queen's University, Kingston, ON, Canada

© Springer Nature Switzerland AG 2021   77
J. Gahagan, M. K. Bryson (eds.), *Sex- and Gender-Based Analysis in Public Health*, https://doi.org/10.1007/978-3-030-71929-6_6

rates include tobacco use, alcohol use, exposure to environmental pollution, infections, occupational exposure to known carcinogens and radiation. While the public health efforts to date have largely focused on raising awareness of 'preventable' causes of cancer, this focus tends to offer an emphasis on 'modifiable', individual-level behavioural considerations rather than system-level responses. Over time, countries with sufficient health and cancer care resources have developed risk-based cancer screening programs and systems to address various determinants of health that are regarded as non-modifiable, such as age, race, family history and genetic factors. Not addressed, however, are the broader social and cultural gender-based factors which are less amenable to behaviour change at the level of the individual. In addition, these approaches to cancer prevention often fail to take into account the broader gendered nature of cancer 'risk' or determinants of cancer such as income, income inequality, social capital, social roles, (un)employment and other gender-mediated social factors that can contribute to the pathways that determine health outcomes, including cancer outcomes. This longstanding gender-blind approach is a particularly concerning issue in that approaches to cancer health and care that uncritically deploy the 'women's cancers' moniker of tend to overlook the diversity of experiences of cancers among both older and younger sexual minority and/or gender nonconforming populations such as lesbian, bisexual and transgender populations (Jain, 2007; Kamen et al., 2015; Taylor et al., 2019; Rail et al. 2018). How we understand cancer risk, screening and treatment requires further interrogation within public health practices to ensure a more nuanced approach to cancer care program development and implementation as a whole.

Sex- and Gender-Based Considerations

The problematizing of cancer 'risk' through the lens of both sex and gender as distinct yet intersecting determinants of health requires us to look beyond the binary conceptualizations of these terms. The key to this is a thorough understanding of the many intersectional approaches to gender in relation to cancer risk and cancer care. With this expanded knowledge comes an evidence-based analysis of how cancer prevention, screening and treatment approaches are impacted by the systemic (mis) understandings of sex, gender, and the many intersectional contributors to these determinants of cancer health and experiences of cancer-health decision-making.

Biological sex is represented as a primary driver for 'women's cancers' and related communications and screening initiatives that, rather than being based on particular anatomical elements such as breast, cervical or ovarian cancers, are by contrast frequently narrated in relation to a very rigid linkage of female sex as determinative of just one gender identity – 'woman'. A person's actual gender identity and expression, however, may obscure the need for cancer screening. Transgender people assigned female at birth, and who do not identify as 'women' may, for example, be overlooked in programs for breast or gynaecologic cancers. This oversight would particularly impact individuals with a family history of one or more particular cancers (e.g. breast) specific to anatomy but frequently overlooked in the depiction of the intended target for cancer screening for 'women's cancers'.

Despite this growing recognition, many national and provincial cancer screening messages, interventions and programs – including cancer registries – tend to overlook this distinction in their campaigns. By presenting their data and screening frameworks in terms of biological sex-based cancer risk, the disseminated information is represented and narrated through the lens of cisnormativity (e.g. gender expression and biological sex are congruent). This approach may result in gender diverse populations remaining absent from the public health cancer prevention, care and treatment discourses as their lack of participation leads to uncaptured data. Further, this may lead to avoidance of cancer screening and care among gender diverse populations who do not see themselves represented in cancer prevention campaigns. Members of sexual or gender minority groups may fear discrimination within hetero- and cis-normative cancer care settings.

Approaches to Incorporating Sex- and Gender-Based Analysis (SGBA) in Cancer Care

The following section offers an overview of examples of how sex- and gender-based analysis (SGBA) has been used in cancer care with a focus on how this can be used in public health practice. As indicated by the Canadian Institutes of Health Research (CIHR), the concept of 'sex' 'refers to a set of biological attributes in humans and animals. It is primarily associated with physical and physiological features including chromosomes, gene expression, hormone levels and function, and reproductive/sexual anatomy. Sex is generally categorized as female or male but there is variation in the biological attributes that comprise sex and how those attributes are expressed' (CIHR, 2015). 'Gender', however, depending on the use ,of the term, is both an individual and societal concept. It refers to 'the socially constructed roles, behaviours, expressions and identities of girls, women, boys, men, and gender diverse people. It influences how people perceive themselves and each other, how they act and interact, and the distribution of power and resources in society. Gender is usually conceptualized as a binary (girl/woman and boy/man) yet there is considerable diversity in how individuals and groups understand, experience, and express it' (CIHR, 2015).

In addition to this, it is important to note that cancer registries do not offer more nuanced approaches to data collection, for example, by designing methods to collect demographic data inclusive of gender-diverse populations. This is problematic in that it reduces the specificity of data collected on rates of cancer as well as cancer survival rates for gender diverse populations. The ways in which cancer data are collected remains an important systems-level issue which needs to be reconsidered in an effort to address the failure of current cancer care approaches in meeting the cancer care needs of sexual and gender-diverse cancer patient populations.

To the best of our knowledge, our 'Cancer's Margins' project (www.lgbtcancer.ca) is the first nationally funded, transnational study to document gynaecologic and breast cancer knowledge pathways in relation to minority sexuality – queer, lesbian, bisexual people – and minority gender identity and expression: two-spirit, gender diverse and transgender people (Bryson et al., 2019). For this project, we interviewed a diverse group made up of 81 LBQ (lesbian, bisexual, queer) and/or T2S (transgender or two-spirit) people diagnosed and treated for gynaecologic and/or breast cancers.

The analysis of the patient interviews showed that minority stress and the enduring stigma linked with sexual and/or gender minority cancer patients' histories of discrimination and relatedly, facing systematic and provider-related barriers to adequate care, significantly impacted experiences of cancer care communications and contexts. Our interviewees' cancer experience narratives provide documentation of a strong relationship between perceptions of cultural safety and experiences of sexual and/or gender minority cancer patients. In particular, decisions about interviewees' disclosures about gender identity and/or sexuality were directly linked with perceptions of safety and the possible impact of disclosure on the quality of cancer care.

Trans and gender-diverse as well as two-spirit (T2S) interviewees accounts of cancer health and care experiences frequently included evidence that people, whose gender identity does not easily map onto the intended recipients of cancer health interventions such as cancer screening, were denied care or were provided care in a manner that did not appropriately address their actual gender identity. For T2S interviewees, particular cancer surgeries, such as mastectomy or hysterectomy, were in fact experienced as gender-affirming healthcare – these surgical procedures are, after all, very similar procedures that can form a key aspect of female-assigned T2S gender-affirming care protocols. A particular problem for T2S cancer patients was the complete disconnect between gender-affirming healthcare protocols that include the administration of hormones, with these cancer patients' cancer health care.

Sexual and gender minority cancer patients whom we interviewed faced effects of compounding marginalization that contributed to social isolation and barriers to accessing cancer support groups. This effect was particularly deleterious for gender minority participants in our study, who had less family and friend support compared with cisgender cancer patients (Taylor & Bryson, 2016).

While there is significant room for improvement in relation to cancer prevention, screening, treatment and surveillance, there is a movement toward public health initiatives that are being designed from an SGBA perspective to address this gap in care provision. In the Canadian context, a prime example of this is Cancer Care Ontario's implementation of their 2019 policy 'Overarching Policy for the Screening of Trans People in the Ontario Breast Screening Program and the Ontario Cervical Screening Program'. This policy is meant to address the lack of evidence-based guidelines for screening transgender persons in either the Ontario Breast Screening Program (OBSP) and the Ontario Cervical Screening Program (OCSP) (Carpenter & Broeckaert, 2019). To develop this policy, Cancer Care

Ontario first created five evidence-based products regarding cancer care for transgender people based on a review of the literature, a combination of national and international policies and jurisdictional scans. Two evidence-based products were developed to address cervical cancer screening: Cervical Screening for Transgender Populations: A Guidelines Review and Benefits, Performance and Harms of Cervical Cancer Screening for the Transgender Population: A Systematic Review. Three evidence-based products were developed to address breast cancer screening, in this population: Breast Cancer Screening for Transgender Populations: A Guideline Review; Effectiveness, Benefits and Harms of Breast Cancer Screening for the Transgender Population: A Systematic Review; and Breast Cancer Risk, Prognosis, and Mortality in the Transgender Population Using Cross-Sex Hormones: A Systematic Review (Carpenter & Broeckaert, 2019). These publications were then assessed by two expert working groups who provided their clinical recommendations to the steering committee, which then reviewed the clinical recommendations. This process led to an evidence-based, peer-reviewed set of recommendations for the OBSP and OCSP programs regarding the screening of transgender persons. It is important to note is that the steering committee was comprised not only of medical professionals but also included members of the transgender community.

Beyond their clinical recommendations, the authors of this policy also identified public health system barriers to its implementation in Ontario. At the policy level, it was identified that there are some services listed in the recommendations that, for example, are not currently available through the OBSP and OCSP; the authors note that forthcoming updates to the screening to programs will align with the recommendations (Carpenter & Broeckaert, 2019). Looking at the policy implementation level, it was found that as the screening program notification process is dependent on sex designation, there was the potential for transgender individuals who would qualify for the screening program based on biology, but not receive notifications. For example, due to the conflation of the concepts of sex and gender in the design of the Ontario Health Insurance Plan (OHIP) registry, a transgender male patient with a cervix would not receive OCSP correspondence if their OHIP file was changed to match their gender identity of male. At the care provision level, primary care provider billing codes that allow for certain tests to be sent to the lab and processed, as well as allowing the physician to be recompensed for the procedure to acquire the sample, are formatted based on sex designation. For example, when a transgender man with a cervix has a Pap smear, this test could be rejected as their sex marker 'M' would not align with the accepted female sex marker 'F' in the Pap smear billing code.

Given this, it is not only a case of policy development and implementation, but the entire public health system also must take up the challenge of implementing comprehensive gender-transformative care in cancer prevention, screening and treatment. It is a combination of the system, the policy and the knowledge of care providers that must act synergistically to effect positive change for the lives of LGBTQ+ persons diagnosed with cancer, or engaging with public health systems designed to enhance cancer prevention or detection.

Conclusion

This chapter provides an overview of key issues in relation to how sex and gender synergistically and intersectionally contribute to cancer prevention, screening and care for those who are assigned female at birth. Key take-away messages for public health practitioners – including those in epidemiological surveillance, clinical care and in training/teaching roles in cancer care – is the need for greater emphasis on both the sex and gendered nature of cancer risk, as well as the importance of differentiating the two concepts in cancer programs and policies. It is this differentiation that will allow public health cancer care systems to provide health-affirming, patient-centred policies and approaches in cancer care provision. The importance of this distinction can be found in the lack of data in cancer registries that consider sex and gender as concepts that are not static but rather may be fluid across the life course in understanding cancer incidence, prevalence and outcomes.

Developing gender-transformative cancer care requires public health systems to support the design and implementation of cancer screening approaches that address systemic barriers to cancer care such as transphobia and homophobia in cancer screening policy directives, as well as in epidemiological studies and cancer registries. For example, available data on rates of breast cancer shows higher incidence among lesbians, and yet despite this, we know that lesbians are often reluctant to engage with formal healthcare systems, including cancer screening services, due to homophobia inherent in such systems. This is further compounded for transgender men and other gender nonconforming populations who may not be offered screening for 'women's cancers' despite a known family history and other risk factors for breast cancer. Gender-transformative cancer screening for lesbian, bisexual and transgender populations must, therefore, address gender-based inequalities that can prevent uptake of cancer screening programs by practitioners and barriers to buy-in from patients.

References

Bryson, M., Taylor, E., Boschman, L., Hart, T., Gahagan, J., Rail, G., & Ristock, J. (2019). Awkward choreographies from cancer's margins: Incommensurabilities of biographical and biomedical knowledge in sexual and/or gender minority cancer patients' treatment. *Journal of Medical Humanities, 40*(2), 1–21.

Burkhalter, J. E., Margolies, L., Sigurdsson, H. O., Walland, J., Radix, A. E., Rice, D., & Maingi, S. (2016). The national LGBT cancer action plan: A white paper of the 2014 national summit on cancer in the LGBT communities. *LGBT Health, 3*(1), 19–31.

Carpenter, B., & Broeckaert, L. (2019). *Overarching policy for the screening of trans people in the Ontario breast screening program and the Ontario cervical screening program.* Cancer Care Ontario. Available online. https://www.cancercareontario.ca/sites/ccocancercare/files/guidelines/full/Policy_ScreeningTransPeopleOBSPandOXCSP.pdf. Accessed 12 Jan 2020.

Canadian Institutes of Health Research. (2015). *Definitions of sex and gender.* https://cihr-irsc.gc.ca/e/47830.html. Accessed Aug 2019.

Jain, S. (2007). Cancer butch. *Cultural Anthropology, 22*(4), 501–538.

Kamen, C. S., Smith-Stoner, M., Heckler, C., Flannery, M., & Margolies, L. (2015). Social support, self-rated health, and lesbian, gay, bisexual, and transgender identity disclosure to cancer care providers. *Oncology Nursing Forum, 42*(1), 44–51.

Rail, G., Molina, L., Fusco, C., Norman, M., Petherick, L., Moola, F., & Bryson, M. (2018). HPV vaccination discourses and the construction of "at-risk" girls. *Canadian Journal of Public Health., 109*(5–6), 622–621.

Sulik, A. (2011). *Pink ribbon blues: How breast cancer culture undermines women's health.* New York, NY: Oxford University Press.

Taylor, E., Bryson, M., Boschman, L., Hart, T., Gahagan, J., Rail, G., & Ristock, J. (2019). Cancer's margins: Knowledge ecologies, access to knowledge, and knowledge mobilization by sexual and/or gender minority cancer patients. *Media and Communication, 7*(1), 102–113.

Taylor, E., & Bryson, M. (2016). Cancer's Margins: Trans and gender nonconforming people's access to knowledge, experiences of cancer health, and decision-making. *LGBT Health., 3*(1), 1–11.

WHO. (2018). https://www.who.int/cancer/prevention/en/

Chapter 7
Tuberculosis and the Relevance of Sex- and Gender-Based Analysis

Sizulu Moyo, Olanrewaju Oladimeji, Jeremiah Chikovore, and Nompumelelo Zungu

Global TB Burden

Tuberculosis (TB) is an airborne disease that is caused by the *Mycobacterium tuberculosis (M.tb) bacilli*. It remains the leading cause of significant morbidity and mortality globally, despite concerted global effort to reduce its burden (Kyu et al., 2017; WHO, 2018a). In 2017, there were 10 million new cases of TB and 1.6 million deaths from the disease (WHO, 2018a). Although TB affects people in all countries, the TB burden varies across countries and regions. In 2017, there were less than 10 new TB cases/100,000 population in most high-income countries, 150–400/100,000 in most of the 30 high TB burden countries, and above 500/100,000 new cases in a few countries including Mozambique, the Philippines, and South Africa. Three per cent (3%) of new cases were in the World Health Organization (WHO) European Region and 3% in the WHO Region of the Americas

S. Moyo (✉)
Human Sciences Research Council, Human and Social Capabilities Programme, Cape Town, South Africa

School of Public Health, University of Cape Town, Cape Town, South Africa
e-mail: smoyo@hsrc.ac.za

O. Oladimeji
Department of Global Health and Population, Harvard T.H. Chan School of Public Health, Boston, MA, USA

J. Chikovore
Human and Social Capabilities Research Division, Human Sciences Research Council, Durban, South Africa

N. Zungu
Human Sciences Research Council, Pretoria, South Africa

Department of Psychology, University of Pretoria, Pretoria, South Africa

© Springer Nature Switzerland AG 2021
J. Gahagan, M. K. Bryson (eds.), *Sex- and Gender-Based Analysis in Public Health*, https://doi.org/10.1007/978-3-030-71929-6_7

(WHO, 2018a). Men, people living in Asia and Africa, and those living with HIV are the most affected by TB (Floyd et al., 2018; Horton et al., 2016; Rhines, 2013; WHO, 2018a). In 2017, eight Asian and African countries accounted for about two-thirds of the global TB burden, 90% of all new TB cases occurred in adults (≥15 years), and 9% in people living with HIV, (WHO, 2018a). Trends in incident TB cases between 2000 and 2017 show a slow decline in the global TB burden (WHO, 2018a).

TB Burden by Sex and Age

TB data is generally disaggregated by sex, and TB prevalence surveys and TB notifications have shown a higher burden of TB among men across all geographic regions with about two-thirds of all TB notifications coming from men (Borgdorff et al., 2000; Holmes et al., 1998; Horton et al., 2016). The male-to-female TB prevalence ratio in the Africa region has increased over time, and the higher prevalence among males has remained persistent even in countries with generalized HIV epidemics and a higher HIV prevalence among females, (Horton et al., 2016). The difference in the male and female TB burden is thought to be partially mediated by male and female genetic differences and by differences in the immune response that is influenced by sex hormones (Nhamoyebonde & Leslie, 2014). Consistent with the higher burden in men, global TB mortality statistics indicate a consistently higher TB mortality in men compared to women (WHO, 2018a).

The broad disaggregation of TB data by sex that shows a higher burden in men, however, this masks significant epidemiological differences in some regions and in some age groups. These differences have important public health and policy implications in relation to the need for sex- and gender-based analysis of data and related relevant programmatic responses. For example, in some areas of Afghanistan, Pakistan, and Iran the burden of TB is higher in females (WHO, 2018b). Furthermore, women in the reproductive age group bear a significant burden of TB, with up to 10% of maternal mortality attributable to TB (WHO, 2018b).

Data has also shown differences in the TB burden by age, with young children especially those less than 2 years old at the greatest risk of TB (Marais et al., 2004). Thereafter, the burden of TB increases with age from adolescence consistent with reactivation of latent infection in the presence of weakened immunity due to other infections or older age. Data from low-and middle-income countries showed an increase in the male-to-female prevalence ratio of TB with age from 1.28 in individuals aged 15–24 years to 3.18 in individuals aged 45–54 years (Horton et al., 2016). A study in Nigeria reported the largest sex differences in the distribution of TB in those younger than 30 years old; males aged 25–29 years had a higher burden of TB infection, while females in the same age group have a higher burden of TB-HIV (Aliyu et al., 2018).

TB and Pregnancy

While overall TB mortality is greater in men, TB is a leading cause of mortality among women in the reproductive age group (Adhikari, 2009; Ahmed et al., 1999; Grange et al., 2010; Mathad & Gupta, 2012). This is related to untreated TB in pregnancy being as high as 40% (Adhikari, 2009; Mathad & Gupta, 2012). The effects of TB on pregnancy are influenced by the severity of the TB, the stage of the pregnancy, and the presence of other comorbidities (Bates et al., 2015). HIV is potentially the most significant comorbidity in this regard with over 50% (Khan et al., 2001) of TB maternal mortality caused by HIV. Frequent and consecutive pregnancies promote reactivation of latent TB and TB in pregnancy can be more difficult to detect and diagnose, since the clinical picture is nonspecific. For example, weight loss due to TB could be masked by the weight gain caused by the pregnancy. Therefore, without a high index of suspicion and awareness among clinicians, pregnant women with TB can easily be missed leading to diagnostic delays and poor treatment outcomes (Sulis & Pai, 2018). Undiagnosed and untreated TB in pregnancy may be transmitted to the baby in utero or postnatally, with the baby needing special treatment and care that the mother might not be able to administer if she herself is ill from TB. Women also have a greater risk of extrapulmonary TB, including genital TB, which can result in infertility (Chavhan et al., 2004; Thorson & Diwan, 2001; WHO, 2002), with significant consequences for many women in high TB settings. Therefore, it is important that TB data be disaggregated by sex, age, geographic area, socioeconomic, and other locally relevant variables in order to implement appropriate mitigation strategies.

TB and HIV

HIV is the most significant TB comorbidity in high TB burden settings, with HIV fuelling the TB epidemic. Being HIV positive significantly increases the risk of developing TB. People living with HIV are 26–31 times more likely to develop TB than those without HIV, with the greatest impact being on pregnant women. TB is also the most common presenting illness among people living with HIV, even among those on antiretroviral treatment, and it remains a major cause of HIV-related deaths (Bates et al., 2015; WHO, 2018b). While HIV especially in Western countries was initially higher among gay males, it is now much higher among women, and many high HIV burden countries have higher rates of new HIV infections in young women (UNAIDS, 2018). With these high rates of HIV, these women have an increased risk of TB in general, and this is exacerbated by pregnancy (Khan et al., 2001). In Nigeria, TB-HIV coinfection was highest in females aged 25–29 years (Aliyu et al., 2018), the age group where women are known to have high rates of HIV incidence.

Socio-Cultural Norms

The higher burden of TB in men is partly driven by social and cultural norms in that TB is an airborne disease and transmission occurs in crowded and poorly ventilated spaces. In many cultures, men generally work outside the home, tend to socialize more outside the home, have more social contacts (UNDP, 2015), and thereby increase their risk of acquiring TB given its mode of transmission. TB in men is also partly driven by the gender-specific occupations in which men are more likely than women to work such as in mines where mineworkers have a greater risk and burden of TB. Tobacco use and alcohol intake are well-known risk factors for TB, and men are more likely to use tobacco and alcohol, contributing to their higher risk and burden of TB. However, it is now common for women to work outside the home in many settings, and hence, they are also exposed to some of the same risk factors as men. Furthermore, men who acquire TB at work or in social settings transmit it to women in their homes, thereby influencing the risk and burden of TB in these women. Data also shows that more women have been taking up smoking and this undoubtedly increases their risk of TB. Therefore, without detailed sex- and gender-based analysis of occupational TB data, interventions would exclude these women who are also at increased risk of TB.

Education and Knowledge about TB

TB education and knowledge dissemination through various awareness platforms remain key components of achieving effective TB control and elimination. The literature presents a mixed picture on TB knowledge by sex: - some studies show similar levels of knowledge (Cramm et al., 2010; Mfinanga et al., 2008; Westaway, 1989; Zuma et al., 2016), some show higher levels of TB knowledge in men (Marks et al., 2008; Naidoo et al., 2016; Promtussananon & Peltzer, 2005; Weiss et al., 2008), and others show the opposite (Deribew et al., 2010; Hoa et al., 2009; Karim et al., 2007; Zhang et al., 2007). Data from South Africa showed that being male, being of mixed race, being employed, and learning about TB from the television, brochures, and healthcare workers were associated with higher levels of TB knowledge (Naidoo et al., 2016). Still, in South Africa, 14.6% of adults ≥15 years (14.2% males and 14.9% females) enrolled in an HIV prevalence survey conducted in 2017 incorrectly reported that TB was always linked to HIV, with 11% of respondents reporting that they did not have any knowledge about this (10% each in males and females) (Simbayi et al., 2019). Improving community knowledge about TB is critical and helps to improve health-seeking behaviour (Khan et al., 2001; Bam et al., 2014).

Healthcare-Seeking and Access to Health Services

The WHO recommends that countries with high burdens of TB adopt and ensure universal and free access to TB services. This is to enable all individuals with TB to be diagnosed and treated early (Dara et al., 2016; Migliori et al., 2018; Sotgiu et al., 2016), since early detection and treatment of TB are essential in disrupting the transmission of infection. It is, however, important to note that while TB treatment might be free, money is often required to pay for transport to healthcare facilities that are not within walking distance. Surveys that examined costs faced by TB patients and their households in Ghana and Kenya found that non-medical costs accounted for the largest share of all costs associated with TB care (WHO, 2018a). In many high TB burden countries, women are often financially dependent on males, and thus, they may not be able to access care as they wish or when they need it (Diwan & Thorson, 2001; Onifade et al., 2010; Oshi et al., 2016). Furthermore, women's health is sometimes viewed as of lower priority, thus limiting women's ability to seek care in a timely manner (Onifade et al., 2010). This, in turn, leads to diagnostic and treatment delays and to women presenting with advanced TB disease (Oshi et al., 2016; WHO, 2017). In addition, the gendered nature of women's roles results in being assigned to caregiving roles for children and the elderly, (Oshi et al., 2016), and these responsibilities affect their ability to seek care if there is no one else available to take over these roles. Women are also the primary caregivers of those with TB within and outside their homes (Crampin et al., 2004), and this increases their risk of contracting TB and of transmitting it to others and in particular to young children (Beyers et al., 1997).

Men, on the other hand, might delay seeking care or opt out of care for different reasons, some of which are gendered in nature. These can include travel for work opportunities, being unable to attend healthcare facilities that do not open beyond regular office hours (Onifade et al., 2010; van den Hof et al., 2010), and other men's gender roles and expectations in their families and communities. Qualitative research from Malawi (Chikovore et al., 2014; Chikovore et al., 2015), for instance, revealed how men internalize or are expected to display concepts of manhood such as being able to provide adequately for their families or possessing abundant assets and resources, while in reality limited opportunities to earn an income makes this unattainable, leaving the men facing social devaluation. The men's response – consistent with some research that has documented the impacts of toxic masculinity on health – is to make concerted efforts to demonstrate these elusive images, even if this involves going to extremes. They may thus avoid seeking care for TB symptoms to escape a diagnosis of TB, because it is perceived to be an incapacitating and serious illness that prevents men from fending for themselves and their families, or because it is perceived to be a disease of women. Men also tend to prioritize work and social activities above seeking care for their symptoms as part of reaffirming their male gender roles and demonstrating that they are still in control of their lives (Chikovore et al., 2014; Mavhu et al., 2010).

A systematic review on barriers and delays in TB diagnosis and treatment services by Yang and colleagues (Yang et al., 2014) found mixed evidence of provider or system-level barriers by gender. Of the 19 studies on provider- or system-level barriers that were analysed 42% showed that women faced greater barriers to accessing TB services. Women in the Gambia saw more healthcare providers before obtaining a TB diagnosis than men (Lienhardt et al., 2001), while in Vietnam, women took more health-seeking actions for their symptoms than men did but were offered sputum smear examinations significantly less often (Thorson et al., 2000).

Gendered social norms also affect the manner in which males and females are treated in healthcare facilities. A lack of privacy can deter both males and females from accessing or remaining in care for TB. Men fear being emasculated at healthcare facilities, in the presence of women and children, if they attend crowded health facilities, or if healthcare workers address them discourteously (Chikovore et al., 2014; Chikovore et al., 2015). Women have also expressed concern about the layout of most health establishments that limit privacy at the point of delivery of DOTS therapy (Onifade et al., 2010).

In the review by Yang and colleagues, 10 of the 22 studies on provider/system level delays found longer delays in women when compared to men. There was a longer presentation to treatment delay and diagnosis to treatment delay in women than in men (Yang et al., 2014). In the Midlands area of the United Kingdom, women TB patients spent 6% more time than males before receiving treatment (Sultan et al., 2013). In Australia, males underwent a chest X-ray or CT scan sooner, began treatment sooner after presentation, and were more likely to have a sputum smear sample performed than women (Dale et al., 2017). Delay in TB diagnosis and initiation of treatment is one of the main factors contributing to the spread of *M.tb* and preventing the elimination of TB.

Treatment Outcomes

Treatment outcomes, categorized as cured, treatment completed, treatment failed, died, loss to follow up, not evaluated, and treatment success, are key indicators of the TB programme. These indicators are monitored to track the TB epidemic at local, national, and international levels (WHO, 2018a). Treatment success is one of the top ten indicators for monitoring implementation of the End TB strategy (WHO, 2015). Men have been reported to have more severe disease and lower smear and culture conversion rates (Dale et al., 2017; Feng et al., 2012). Overall, males have a greater risk of unsuccessful treatment outcomes (Dale et al., 2017; Khatri & Frieden, 2000; WHO, 2002), and more males die from TB. Despite facing more socioeconomic and cultural adversities that affect access to and the quality of care, women on TB treatment tend to have outcomes that are more favourable, suggesting that once women access care they do well.

Stigma

Goffman defines stigma as "an attribute that is deeply discrediting," and that transforms the person it is inflicted upon "from a whole and usual person to a tainted, discounted one" (Goffman, 1963). People with chronic infectious diseases such as TB and HIV still suffer stigma in many communities (Jaramillo et al., 2017; Karim et al., 2007). TB stigma is one of the most important barriers to fighting the TB epidemic (Coleman et al., 2010), and the United Nations agencies have called for an end to discrimination in health care settings (WHO and UNAIDS, 2017). Stigma is characterized by shame, exaggerated fear of transmission, the experience of social exclusion, being discriminated against due to the illness, being made fun of or insulted, and fear of disclosure (Bond, 2011; Bond & Nyblade, 2006; Miller et al., 2017; Weiss, 2008). Understanding the nature of TB stigma and measuring its magnitude are essential components of an effective TB response (Jaramillo et al., 2017).

In regions where HIV and AIDS are endemic, TB-related stigma is intertwined with HIV-related stigma and the intersection of the two types of stigma and the associated discrimination become a critical barrier to the utilization of TB and HIV services by both men and women. HIV stigma also fuels TB stigma in TB-HIV syndemic settings (Bond & Nyblade, 2006; Rood et al., 2017). In many instances, an HIV diagnosis may follow a TB diagnosis, with those diagnosed with TB then subjected to speculations about their HIV status (Møller & Erstad, 2007). TB stigma also intersects with cultural norms, gender roles, and traditional beliefs about what causes the disease and how it is transmitted (Horton et al., 2016; Miller et al., 2017).

The most common cause of TB stigma is the perceived risk of transmission from TB-infected individuals to other members of the community. TB is also stigmatized because of its associations with poverty, lower social class, malnutrition, or perceived disreputable behaviour. TB stigma is therefore influenced by, and may worsen, preexisting gender- and class-based health disparities.

Although both men and women are affected by TB stigma, the literature suggests that TB stigma has more impact on women than on men (van den Hof et al., 2010), as TB is often seen as a disease of women in some cultures (Miller et al., 2017). In Tanzania, TB patients and family members of TB patients reported that women with TB were assumed to be promiscuous and to practice infidelity (by those who believed TB to be a sexually transmitted disease), while some women were divorced by their husbands because they had TB (Miller et al., 2017). For men, TB stigma is reported to result in patients being neglected by family members and being left without food and other support (Miller et al., 2017). Men may also be viewed as having lost control of their lives, and thus unable to provide for their families (Chikovore et al., 2014; Chikovore et al., 2015).

Those with TB symptoms and TB patients also experience stigma when they access care, with reports of bad or poor treatment by healthcare workers (Miller et al., 2017). Research indicates that "providing inferior health care to persons diagnosed with stigmatized conditions such as TB or HIV infection or subjecting them to unnecessary procedures or pain, are common forms of "enacted stigma" in health settings (Straetemans et al., 2017). Stigma within the healthcare setting can also present in subtle forms such as behavioural manifestations of disdain or disgust towards a stigmatized individual, avoidance and distrust by healthcare workers, and verbal micro-aggression.

Summary and SGBA implications in Public Health

The available evidence clearly indicates that sex and gender synergistically influence both the spread of TB as well as TB control. Socially embedded gender roles of both men and women have a significant impact on the risk of developing TB, the burden of TB, access to care, the quality of care, TB stigma, and health outcomes. The population groups that are at greater risk of TB are often also at higher risk for health disparities. It is therefore imperative to understand the sex and gender inequalities in TB by disaggregating key TB indicators using a sex- and gender-based analytical framework that unpacks how sex, gender, and other variables including age, socioeconomic status, and geographic location impact public health responses. This will help to identify where, when, and what inequalities exist and therefore inform appropriate and equitable policies and other interventions. For example, WHO and the United States Agency for International Development (USAID) have recommended that TB data collection and reporting forms at the district level include TB case registration by sex and age. This will help to improve the overall impact of TB programmes and to ensure that women and men of different ages have equitable access to health services.

While some progress is being made, there is still a need for greater efforts to include and be explicit about sex and gender in public health research projects to uncover and address hidden variations in disease burden (Vissandjee et al., 2016). In many research publications and surveillance data, TB outcomes are often not reported disaggregated by sex and where they are, there are often assumptions of homogeneity in the descriptions of women's and men's challenges. Such analyses and presentations of TB data do not take into account the variations in gender relations and gendered hierarchies by context, within and between countries, and the evolution of cultural and social practices and norms over time (Allotey & Gyapong, 2005). In addition, researchers do not always use consistent terminology, making it difficult to identify research with a sex or gender focus and for researchers and policy-makers to access and use such information to address gender-related issues and challenges within TB programs (Vissandjee et al., 2016).

Recommendations

Tuberculosis (TB) remains a leading cause of mortality globally and particularly in low- and middle-income countries. Evidence consistently shows that the burden of TB differs by sex, gender, economic, and other sociodemographic factors. In this chapter, we have highlighted why TB research should include a focus on sex and gender with researchers supported to define and operationalize sex and gender in relation to their studies. It is clear that to address the impacts of gender norms and biases as these affect TB health and care, data regarding TB prevalence and intervention effects should be disaggregated by sex, gender, and other variables within the sex and gender framework such as age, socioeconomic status, and geographic location. There is a need for consistent use of terminology relating to sex and gender to enable public health workers and policy-makers to access and utilize the data to inform TB health monitoring and treatment activities appropriately. Understanding and reporting TB with a consideration of these factors is critical to ensure equity in addressing the TB disease burden with appropriate strategies. Abundant evidence supports the conclusion that there is a need to monitor gender-sensitive indicators that track underlying gender norms and expectations that drive inequalities in TB incidence and outcomes. Therefore, there remains a need for detailed sex- and gender-based analysis of TB at various levels and within local contexts in order to inform strategies that will be effective in supporting the public health goal of ending TB by 2035.

References

Adhikari, M. (2009). Tuberculosis and tuberculosis/HIV co-infection in pregnancy. *Seminars in Fetal & Neonatal Medicine, 14*(4), 234–240.

Ahmed, Y., Mwaba, P., Chintu, C., Grange, J. M., Ustianowski, A., & Zumla, A. (1999). A study of maternal mortality at the University Teaching Hospital, Lusaka, Zambia: The emergence of tuberculosis as a major non-obstetric cause of maternal death. *The International Journal of Tuberculosis and Lung Disease, 3*, 675–680.

Aliyu, G., El-Kamary, S. S., Abimiku, A., Blattner, W., & Charurat, M. (2018). Demography and the dual epidemics of tuberculosis and HIV: Analysis of cross-sectional data from Sub-Saharan Africa. *PLoS One, 13*(9), e0191387. https://doi.org/10.1371/journal.pone.0191387

Allotey, P., & Gyapong, M. (2005). *The gender agenda in the control of tropical diseases: A review of current evidence. Special Topics in Social, Economic and Behavioural (SEB) Research. TDR/STR/SEB/ST/05.1(4).* Geneva: WHO.

Bam, K., Bhatt, L. P., Hapa, R., Dossajee, H. K., & Angdembe, M. R. (2014). Illness perception of tuberculosis (TB) and health seeking practice among urban slum residents of Bangladesh: A qualitative study. *BMC Research, 7*, 572.

Bates, M., Ahmed, Y., Kapata, N., Maeurer, M., Mwaba, P., & Zumla, A. (2015). Perspectives on tuberculosis in pregnancy. *International Journal of Infectious Diseases, 32*, 124–127.

Beyers, N., Gie, R. P., Schaaf, H. S., Van Zyl, S., Talent, J. M., Nel, E. D., & Donald, P. R. (1997). A prospective evaluation of children under the age of 5 years living in the same household as adults with recently diagnosed pulmonary tuberculosis. *The International Journal of Tuberculosis and Lung Disease, 1*(1), 38–43.

Bond, V. (2011). Terrains and tuberculosis: The model applied in urgent public health settings. In S. Wallman (Ed.), *The capability of places: Methods for modelling community response to intrusion and change* (pp. 80–110). London: Pluto Press.

Bond, V., & Nyblade, L. (2006). The importance of addressing the unfolding TB-HIV stigma in high HIV prevalence settings. *Journal of Community and Applied Social Psychology, 16*, 452–461.

Borgdorff, M. W., Nagelkerke, N. J. D., Dye, C., & Nunn, P. (2000). Gender and tuberculosis: A comparison of prevalence surveys with notification data to explore sex differences in case detection. *The International Journal of Tuberculosis and Lung Disease, 4*(2), 123–132.

Chavhan, G. B., Hira, P., Rathod, K., Zacharia, T. T., Chawla, A., Badhe, P., & Parmar, H. (2004). Female genital tuberculosis: Hysterosalpingographic appearances. *The British Journal of Radiology, 77*, 164–169.

Chikovore, J., Hart, G., Kumwenda, M., Chipungu, G. A., & Corbett, L. (2015). 'For a mere cough, men must just chew Conjex, gain strength, and continue working'. The provider construction and tuberculosis care-seeking implications in Blantyre, Malawi. *Global Health Action, 8*(1), 26292. https://doi.org/10.3402/gha.v8.26292

Chikovore, J., Hart, G., Kumwenda, M., Chipungu, G. A., Desmond, N., & Corbett, L. (2014). Control, struggle, and emergent masculinities: A qualitative study of men's care-seeking determinants for chronic cough and tuberculosis symptoms in Blantyre, Malawi. *BMC Public Health, 14*(1), 1053.

Coleman, C. H., Jaramillo, E., Reis, A., & Selgelid, M. (2010). *Guidance on ethics of tuberculosis prevention, care and control* (Vol. 38). Geneva: World Health Organization.

Cramm, J. M., Finkenflügel, H. J., Møller, V., & Nieboer, A. P. (2010). TB treatment initiation and adherence in a South African community influenced more by perceptions than by knowledge of tuberculosis. *BMC Public Health, 10*, 72.

Crampin, A. C., Glynn, J. R., Floyd, S., Malema, S. S., Mwinuka, V. K., Ngwira, B. M., Mwaungulu, F. D., Warndorff, D. K., & Fine, P. E. (2004). Tuberculosis and gender: Exploring the patterns in a case control study in Malawi. *The International Journal of Tuberculosis and Lung Disease, 8*(2), 194–203.

Dale, K., Tay, E., Trauer, J. M., Trevan, P., & Denholm, J. (2017). Gender differences in tuberculosis diagnosis, treatment and outcomes in Victoria, Australia, 2002-2015. *The International Journal of Tuberculosis and Lung Disease, 21*(12), 1264–1271. https://doi.org/10.5588/ijtld.17.0338

Dara, M., Solovic, I., Sotgiu, G., D'Ambrosio, L., Centis, R., Goletti, D., Duarte, R., Aliberti, S., De Benedictis, F. M., Bothamley, G., & Schaberg, T. (2016). Call for urgent actions to ensure access to early diagnosis and care of tuberculosis among refugees: Statement of the European Respiratory Society and the European Region of the International Union Against Tuberculosis and Lung Disease. *The European Respiratory Journal, 47*(5), 1345–1347.

Deribew, A., Abebe, G., Apers, L., Jira, C., Tesfaye, M., Shifa, J., Abdisa, A., Woldemichael, K., Deribie, F., Bezabih, M., & Aseffa, A. (2010). Prejudice and misconceptions about tuberculosis and HIV in rural and urban communities in Ethiopia: A challenge for the TB/HIV control program. *BMC Public Health, 10*, 400.

Floyd, K., Glaziou, P., Zumla, A., & Raviglione, M. (2018). The global tuberculosis epidemic and progress in care, prevention, and research: An overview in year 3 of the End TB era. *The Lancet Respiratory Medicine, 6*(4), 299–314.

Goffman, E. (1963). *Stigma: Notes on the management of spoiled identity*. Englewood Cliffs: Prentice Hall.

Grange, J., Adhikari, M., Ahmed, Y., Mwaba, P., Dheda, K., Hoelscher, M., & Zumla, A. (2010). Tuberculosis in association with HIV/AIDS emerges as a major nonobstetric cause of maternal mortality in Sub-Saharan Africa. *International Journal of Gynaecology and Obstetrics, 108*(3), 181–183. https://doi.org/10.1016/j.ijgo.2009.12.005

Hoa, N. P., Chuc, N. T. K., & Thorson, A. (2009). Knowledge, attitudes, and practices about tuberculosis and choice of communication channels in a rural community in Vietnam. *Health Policy, 90*(1), 8–12.

Holmes, C. B., Hausler, H., & Nunn, P. (1998). A review of sex differences in the epidemiology of tuberculosis. *International Journal of Tuberculosis and Lung Diseases, 2*, 96–104.

Horton, K. C., MacPherson, P., Houben, R. M., White, R. G., & Corbett, E. L. (2016). Sex differences in tuberculosis burden and notifications in low- and middle-income countries: A systematic review and meta-analysis. *PLoS Med, 13*(9), e1002119. https://doi.org/10.1371/journal.pmed.1002119

Jaramillo, E., Sahu, S., & Van Weezenbeek, C. (2017). Ending TB-related stigma and discrimination. *The International Journal of Tuberculosis and Lung Disease, 21*(11), S2–S3. https://doi.org/10.5588/ijtld.16.0914

Johansson, E., Long, N. H., Diwan, V. K., & Winkvist, A. (2000). Gender and tuberculosis control: Perspectives on health seeking behaviour among men and women in Vietnam. *Health Policy, 52*(1), 33–51. https://doi.org/10.1016/S0168-8510(00)00062-2

Karim, F., Islam, M. A., Chowdhury, A. M., Johansson, E., & Diwan, V. K. (2007). Gender differences in delays in diagnosis and treatment of tuberculosis. *Health Policy and Planning, 22*, 329–334.

Khan, M., Pillay, T., Moodley, J. M., & Connolly, C. A. (2001). Maternal mortality associated with tuberculosis–HIV-1 co-infection in Durban, South Africa. *AIDS, 15*, 1857–1863.

Khatri, G. R., & Frieden, T. R. (2000). The status and prospectus of tuberculosis control in India. *The International Journal of Tuberculosis and Lung Disease, 4*, 193–200.

Kyu, H. H., Maddison, E. R., Henry, N. J., Mumford, J. E., Barber, R., Shields, C., Brown, J. C., Nguyen, G., Carter, A., Wolock, T. M., & Wang, H. (2017). The global burden of tuberculosis: Results from the Global Burden of Disease Study 2015. *The Lancet Infectious Diseases, 18*(3), 261–284.

Lienhardt, C., Rowley, J., Manneh, K., Lahai, G., Needham, D., Milligan, P., & McAdam, K. P. (2001). Factors affecting time delay to treatment in a tuberculosis control programme in a sub-Saharan African country: The experience of the Gambia. *The International Journal of Tuberculosis and Lung Disease, 5*(3), 233–239.

Marais, B. J., Gie, R. P., Schaaf, H. S., Hesseling, A. C., Obihara, C. C., Starke, J. J., Enarson, D. A., Donald, P. R., & Beyers, N. (2004). The natural history of childhood intra-thoracic tuberculosis: A critical review of literature from the prechemotherapy era. *The International Journal of Tuberculosis and Lung Disease, 8*, 392–402.

Marks, S. M., Deluca, N., & Walton, W. (2008). Knowledge, attitudes and risk perceptions about tuberculosis: US national health interview survey. *The International Journal of Tuberculosis and Lung Disease, 12*(11), 1261–1267.

Mathad, J. S., & Gupta, A. (2012). Tuberculosis in pregnant and postpartum women: Epidemiology, management, and research gaps. *Clinical Infectious Diseases, 55*(11), 1532–1549. https://doi.org/10.1093/cid/cis732

Mavhu, W., Dauya, E., Bandason, T., Munyati, S., Cowan, F. M., Hart, G., Corbett, E. L., & Chikovore, J. (2010). Chronic cough and its association with TB-HIV coinfection: Factors affecting help-seeking behaviour in Harare, Zimbabwe. *Tropical Medicine and International Health, 15*(5), 574–579.

Mfinanga, S. G., Mutayoba, B. K., Kahwa, A., Kimaro, G., Mtandu, R., Ngadaya, E., Egwaga, S., & Kitua, A. Y. (2008). The magnitude and factors associated with delays in management of smear positive tuberculosis in Dar es Salaam, Tanzania. *BMC Health Services Research, 8*, 158.

Migliori, G. B., Sotgiu, G., Rosales-Klintz, S., Centis, R., D'Ambrosio, L., Abubakar, I., Bothamley, G., Caminero, J. A., Cirillo, D. M., Dara, M., & de Vries, G. (2018). ERS/ECDC statement: European Union Standards for Tuberculosis Care, 2017 update. *The European Respiratory Journal, 51*, 1702678.

Miller, C., Huston, J., Samu, L., Mfinanga, S., Hopewell, P., & Fair, E. (2017). 'It makes the patient's spirit weaker': Tuberculosis stigma and gender interaction in Dar es Salaam, Tanzania. *The International Journal of Tuberculosis and Lung Disease, 21*(11), S42–S48. https://doi.org/10.5588/ijtld.16.0914

Møller, V., & Erstad, I. (2007). Stigma associated with tuberculosis in a time of HIV/AIDS: Narratives from the Eastern Cape, South Africa. *South Africa Review of Sociology, 38*, 103–119.

Naidoo, P., Simbayi, L., Labadarios, D., Ntsepe, Y., Bikitsha, N., Khan, G., Sewpaul, R., Moyo, S., & Rehle, T. (2016). Predictors of knowledge about tuberculosis: Results from SANHANES I, a national, cross-sectional household survey in South Africa. *BMC Public Health, 16*, 276. https://doi.org/10.1186/s12889-016-2951-y

Nhamoyebonde, S., & Leslie, A. (2014). Biological differences between the sexes and susceptibility to tuberculosis. *The International Journal of Tuberculosis and Lung Disease, 209*(3), S100–S106. https://doi.org/10.1093/infdis/jiu147

Onifade, D. A., Bayer, A. M., Montoya, R., Haro, M., Alva, J., Franco, J., Sosa, R., Valiente, B., Valera, E., Ford, C. M., & Acosta, C. D. (2010). Gender factors influencing tuberculosis control in shanty towns: A qualitative study. *BMC Public Health, 10*, 381.

Oshi, D. C., Chukwu, J. N., Nwafor, C. C., Meka, A. O., Madichie, N. O., Ogbudebe, C. L., Onyeonoro, U. U., Ikebudu, J. N., Ekckc, N., Anyim, M. C., & Ukwaja, K. N. (2016). Does intensified case finding increase tuberculosis case notification among children in resource-poor settings? A report from Nigeria. *International Journal of Mycobacteriology, 5*, 44–50.

Promtussananon, S., & Peltzer, K. (2005). Perceptions of tuberculosis: Attributions of cause, suggested means of risk reduction, and preferred treatment in the Limpopo province, South Africa. *Journal of Health, Population and Nutrition, 23*(1), 74–81.

Rhines, A. S. (2013). The role of sex differences in the prevalence and transmission of tuberculosis. *Tuberculosis, 93*, 104–107.

Rood, E. J. J., Mergenthaler, C., Bakker, M. I., Redwood, L., & EMH, M. (2017). Using 15 DHS surveys to study epidemiological correlates of TB courtesy stigma and health-seeking behaviour. *The International Journal of Tuberculosis and Lung Disease, 21*(11), S60–S68. https://doi.org/10.5588/ijtld.16.0909

Simbayi, L. C., Zuma, K., Zungu, N., Moyo, S., Marinda, E., Jooste, S., Mabaso, M., Ramlagan, S., North, A., Van Zyl, J., & Mohlabane, N. (2019). *South African national HIV prevalence, incidence, behaviour and communication survey, 2017*. Cape Town: HSRC Press.

Sotgiu, G., Beer, N., Aliberti, S., Migliori, G. B., & Van Der Werf, M. J. (2016). Fighting tuberculosis in the EU/EEA: Towards the new European Union standards on tuberculosis care. *The European Respiratory Journal, 48*, 1278–1281.

Straetemans, M., Bakker, M., & Mitchell, E. (2017). Correlates of observing and willingness to report stigma towards HIV clients by (TB) health workers in Africa. *The International Journal of Tuberculosis and Lung Disease, 21*(11), S6–S18(13).

Sulis, G., & Pai, M. (2018). Tuberculosis in pregnancy: A treacherous yet neglected issue. *Journal of Obstetrics and Gynaecology Canada, 40*(8), 1003–1005. https://doi.org/10.1016/j.jogc.2018.04.041

Sultan, H., Haroon, S., & Syed, N. (2013). Delay and completion of tuberculosis treatment: A cross-sectional study in the west midlands, UK. *Journal of Public Health (Oxford, England), 35*(1), 12–20. https://doi.org/10.1093/pubmed/fds046

Thorson, A., & Diwan, V. K. (2001). Gender inequalities in tuberculosis: Aspects of infection, notification rates, and compliance. *Current Opinion in Pulmonary Medicine, 7*, 165–169.

Thorson, A., Hoa, N. P., & Long, N. H. (2000). Health-seeking behaviour of individuals with a cough of more than 3 weeks. *The Lancet, 356*(9244), 1823–1824.

United Nations Development Programme. (2015). Gender and Tuberculosis. Discussion paper. https://www.aidsdatahub.org/sites/default/files/resource/gender-and-tb-discussion-paper-2015.pdf

UNAIDS. (2018). *UNAIDS data 2018*. Available at http://www.unaids.org/sites/default/files/media_asset/unaids-data-2018_en.pdf

United Nations Development Programme. Gender and Tuberculosis. Discussion paper 2015. https://www.aidsdatahub.org/sites/default/files/resource/gender-and-tb-discussion-paper-2015.pdf

van den Hof, S., Antillon Najlis, C., Bloss, E., & Straetemans, M. (2010). A systematic review on the role of gender in tuberculosis control, challenge TB, *The Hague*, http://www.tbcare1.org/publications/toolbox/tools/access/Role_of_Gender_in_TB_Control.pdf

Vissandjee, B., Mourid, A., Greenaway, C. A., Short, W. E., & Proctor, J. A. (2016). Searching for sex- and gender-sensitive tuberculosis research in public health: Finding a needle in a haystack. *International Journal of Women's Health, 8*, 731–742.

Weiss, M. (2008). Perceptions of gender and tuberculosis in south Indian urban community. *The Indian Journal of Tuberculosis, 55*, 9–14.

Weiss, M. G., Somma, D., Karim, F., Abouihia, A., Auer, C., Kemp, J., & Jawahar, M. S. (2008). Cultural epidemiology of TB with reference to gender in Bangladesh, India and Malawi. *The International Journal of Tuberculosis and Lung Disease, 12*(7), 837–847.

Westaway, M. S. (1989). Knowledge, beliefs and feelings about tuberculosis. *Health Education Research, 4*(2), 205–211.

World Health Organization. (2015). *The END TB strategy*. Geneva: WHO; WHO/HTM/TB/2015.19.
World Health Organization. (2017). *Gender, equity and human rights*. Geneva: WHO.
World Health Organization (WHO). (2002). *Gender and tuberculosis*. Geneva: WHO Department of Gender and Women's Health. Retrieved from http://www.who.int/gender-equity-rights/knowledge/a85584/en/.
World Health Organization (WHO). (2018a). *Global tuberculosis report*. Geneva: World Health Organization; Licence: CC BY-NC-SA 3.0 IGO.
World Health Organization (WHO). (2018b). *TB and Women fact sheet*. Geneva: World Health Organization.
World Health Organization, & UNAIDS. (2017). *Joint United Nations statement on ending discrimination in health care settings 2017*. Available from: http://www.who.int/mediacentre/news/statements/2017/discrimination-in-health-care/en/
Yang, W., Gounder, C. R., Akande, T., De Neve, J. W., KN, M. I., Chandrasekhar, A., de Lima Pereira, A., Gummadi, N., Samanta, S., & Gupta, A. (2014). Barriers and delays in tuberculosis diagnosis and treatment services: Does gender matter? *Tuberculosis Research and Treatment, 2014*, 461935. https://doi.org/10.1155/2014/461935
Zhang, T. H., Liu, X. Y., Bromley, H., & Tang, S. L. (2007). Perceptions of tuberculosis and health seeking behaviour in rural Inner Mongolia, China. *Health Policy, 81*(2–3), 155–165.
Zuma, K., Simbayi, L. C., Rehle, T., Mbelle, N., Zungu, N. P., Mthembu, J., North, A., Van Zyl, J., Jooste, S., Moyo, S., & Wabiri, N. (2016). *The health of our educators in public schools in South Africa*.

Chapter 8
Women, Alcohol and the Public Health Response: Moving Forward from Avoidance, Inattention and Inaction to Gender-Based Design

Nancy Poole

"The temperance movement vilified the saloon as a den of iniquity that sent forth drunkards to impoverish, injure and perhaps murder their families, and drinking establishments of any type were portrayed as the enemies of all women. Women who frequented such places were assumed to be prostitutes or gin-shop derelicts." (p. 76)

Social workers described scene after scene of child neglect due to alcohol. "Drunkenness among the women is ten times worse than in men" stated J.J. Kelso, Ontario's superintendent of neglected and dependent children [in testimony to a Royal Commission in 1893]. "It causes them to lose their maternal instinct and feeling, and they become thoroughly degraded". (p. 82)

"While the medical profession decried the lack of controls over the patent medicine trade, practitioners themselves were guilty of introducing many to alcohol dependency. The middle to late decades of the nineteenth century were the heyday of therapeutic use of alcohol… the dangers of iatrogenically produced alcoholism were real, particularly for women, who most commonly frequently physicians… [In 1880] the Lancet published as series of articles on the medical use of wine by variety and region. The third instalment, for instance, extolled the virtues of red Bordeaux wines." (p. 73)

N. Poole (✉)
Centre of Excellence for Women's Health, Vancouver, BC, Canada

CanFASD Research Network, Vancouver, BC, Canada
e-mail: npoole@cw.bc.ca

© Springer Nature Switzerland AG 2021   99
J. Gahagan, M. K. Bryson (eds.), *Sex- and Gender-Based Analysis in Public Health*, https://doi.org/10.1007/978-3-030-71929-6_8

From "Oh Lord, pour a cordial in her wounded heart": The drinking woman in Victoria and Edwardian Canada. In C. K. Warsh (Ed.), *Drink in Canada, Historical Essays*

Herstory

The eighteenth-century public health discourse about women and alcohol in Canada, as described in *Drink in Canada* (Warsh, 1993), is rich with paternalism. Included in the historical discourse are the criticism of women entering the workforce and drinking in public (the 'fallen woman'), the disparagement of women who drink and neglect their husbands and children (the 'bad mother') and the conflicted role of the medical profession in dispensing of tonics and encouragement of alcohol use while breastfeeding.

Sadly, these threads can still be seen in ongoing public health discourses and approaches regarding women and alcohol, which are characterised by:

- Ambivalence and denial about the rising rates of heavy drinking by women and the health impacts of such consumption. Ann Dowsett Johnson in her recent book *Drink: The intimate relationship between women and alcohol* (Johnston, 2013) captures the story of the rising rates of risky drinking by women and the false linkage to liberation, in the chapter title 'You've come the wrong way baby'.
- Inattention to the prevention of alcohol use in pregnancy and the lack of treatment and support services for mothers with alcohol problems. While fetal alcohol syndrome was reported in the literature in the 1970s, little action on the prevention of alcohol use in pregnancy was put in place until the 1990s. Today, there are moralistic attitudes about women's use of alcohol in pregnancy, exaggeration of the risks (one drink will harm your baby), underestimation of risk and the lack of funding for evidence-based multilevel approaches. There remains no national strategy and scant funding for basic public education on a provincial/territorial or national level.
- Inaction by the healthcare profession in taking up their role in offering brief discussion with all women about the risks of alcohol use and heavy alcohol use. Many current studies discuss how physicians and other health professionals do not feel they have the skills, confidence, time nor required funding to discuss alcohol with women (Holland et al., 2009; Watson et al., 2009), and as a result, screening, brief intervention and referral with women related to alcohol use in pregnancy is not provided universally or systematically. And incorrect advice about the benefits of red wine in breastfeeding also lingers (Crawford-Williams et al., 2015).

So What Does the Public Health Field Need to Attend to, Regarding Alcohol Use by Women?

1. *Prevalence*

The prevalence of alcohol use and alcohol use-related disorders has tended to be higher among boys and men. However, this gender gap appears to be narrowing. Evidence from Canada and the United States reveal a greater increase in rates of alcohol use disorder and binge drinking among women compared with men (White et al., 2015), equally high rates of binge drinking among girls and boys (Cheng et al., 2016) and high rates of alcohol-related hospitalization among young girls (ages 10–19) (Canadian Institute for Health Information, 2017). This is an important shift as alcohol has a more serious impact on girls' and women's health (NIAAA, 2019).

Not all women in Canada and other high-income countries exhibit similar drinking patterns, and so, an intersectional analysis will shed light on important subgroups. There are important risk factors and influences on drinking among women that have not been appropriately incorporated into health promotion efforts. More bisexual (30%) and almost 25% of lesbian women report heavy compared to nearly 15% of heterosexual women (Public Health Agency of Canada, 2018). There are gendered factors that influence drinking by bisexual women such as 'sexual coercion' and 'drinking to cope' (Kelley et al., 2018). These differences in prevalence and patterns of use need to be considered as we start addressing at-risk drinking more effectively. By understanding *which* women are drinking and *why*, we can better devise the support systems and types of information needed to reduce alcohol-related harms. Historically, health promotion efforts have paid little attention to the intersection of gender and other determinants of alcohol use, such as sexuality, race or socioeconomic status.

2. *Key Sex-Related Factors Related to Girls' and Women's Alcohol Use*

Sex-Specific Metabolization of Alcohol   Females tend to have less water in their bodies to dilute the alcohol and less of the enzyme alcohol dehydrogenase, which breaks down alcohol in the stomach. Therefore, females require smaller amounts of alcohol to become intoxicated/reach higher alcohol concentration in the blood (Tuchman, 2010).

Sex-Specific Adverse Health Effects   Since 2004, the National Institute on Alcohol Abuse and Alcoholism in the United States has published reports that document how women who drink alcohol have a higher risk of certain health-related problems. For example, women develop liver cirrhosis with lower quantities of alcohol use (Rehm et al., 2010). Another sex-specific effect has been found through brain imaging, where studies that compare girls and boys with alcohol use disorders report findings which suggest that boys are less sensitive to the neurotoxic effects of alcohol compared to girls. Specifically, girls show a more pronounced reduction in functional brain activation in multiple areas of the brain (Caldwell et al., 2005; Medina et al., 2008). Drinking among women and girls has been connected to breast cancer (Chen et al., 2011; Li et al., 2010), obesity and depression (Farhat et al., 2010; McCarty et al., 2009) and reproductive health problems (Nolen-Hoeksema, 2004). In sum, over the long term, women who drink alcohol are at greater risk of liver damage, heart problems and brain damage than men, and women transition from regular use to alcohol abuse more quickly (NIAAA, 2019). These sex-specific effects of alcohol have implications for (a) what is considered low-risk alcohol use for women, (b) how we report prevalence data, and (c) how we might approach messaging on alcohol and encourage health promotion.

3. *Key Gender-Related Factors Related to Girls' and Women's Alcohol Use*

It is important to examine the influences that account for women's drinking patterns and that illuminate trends by sub-population. However, while the literature often identifies the factors and conditions related to high-risk drinking, the relationships between different factors are not well described and understood, and comprehensive implications for action are seldom drawn.

Alcohol Advertising Alcohol advertising exploits gendered influences on drinking. Jean Kilbourne (1999) has argued that 'alcohol advertising is really our main form of alcohol education'. Young men and women are targeted differently in alcohol advertising, giving women special motives to consume particular brands of alcohol. Journalist Ann Dowsett Johnston has described how the alcohol industry markets directly to girls and young women with beverage names that include the words 'pink' and 'girls' nightout' and beverage flavours that are considered more "feminine" such as kiwi mango (Johnston, 2011). A US study showed girls aged 12–20 years of age were substantially more likely to be exposed to alcohol advertisements than women 21 years and older and girls had 95% more exposure to the cooler or "alcopop "advertising (also called low alcohol refreshers (LAR) even though they contain more alcohol than beer) than women 21 years and older (Jernigan et al., 2004).

Yet while marketing, availability and other influences on use are identified in a recent national report on preventing alcohol and other substance use harms among youth in Canada and some sex-specific prevalence rates mentioned, no gendered approaches to guidelines, school health policies, health warnings, or approaches to reduce access and availability are promoted (Public Health Agency of Canada, 2018).

Alcohol, Pregnancy and Mothering Recognition of the serious, lifelong effects of prenatal alcohol exposure and attention to the prevention of alcohol use in pregnancy could be said to be public health's greatest failure related to women and alcohol. Fetal alcohol spectrum disorders (FASD) is a diagnostic term for the health, learning and social effects that can result from prenatal alcohol exposure, including neurological abnormalities, cognitive and behavioural impairment, minor craniofacial anomalies and birth defects (Chudley et al., 2005; Wozniak et al., 2019). Individuals with FASD will experience some degree of challenges in their daily living and need support with motor skills, physical health, learning, memory, attention, communication, emotional regulation and social skills to reach their full potential (Pei et al., 2019). It is estimated that approximately 10–15% of women do not choose to or are not able to stop drinking alcohol when pregnant (Public Health Agency of Canada, 2009).

Women's reasons for prenatal alcohol and other substance use are complex and gendered. Their substance use is influenced by determinants of health such as experience of abuse, neglect or other forms of trauma, intimate partner violence, physical and mental health concerns, child welfare involvement, poverty and precarious living conditions (Boyd & Marcellus, 2007; Niccols et al., 2010; Pepler et al., 2014). They may have alcohol problems going into the pregnancy, and as such may be more likely to be living with a partner with substance use problems, be isolated and be experiencing lower levels of social support (Marcellus et al., 2014; Sword et al., 2004). Moreover, they are more likely to be stigmatized due to their use, lacking trust towards health and social service providers due to punitive child welfare approaches (Kruk & Banga, 2011) and face other personal, interpersonal and systemic barriers to accessing help. Facing these multiple, interconnected issues can affect women's confidence and capability to seek support, including prenatal health care (Breen et al., 2014; Poole & Isaac, 2001).

A key part of a public health response to women with alcohol concerns is services that are responsive to these multiple health, social, financial, legal and other concerns, where women are offered and can choose the combination of assistance and connections that fit their needs and readiness in an environment of respect and safety. These are important responses for first engagement and, as pathways to ongoing support and other connections for healing, growth and empowerment (Bryans et al., 2012). In Canada, we have the benefit of access to a significant body of public health evidence that documents and assesses service approaches that aim to successfully reach, engage and achieve positive outcomes for pregnant women who use/misuse alcohol: i.e., accessible, women-centred substance use services that are offered in conjunction with prenatal care (Andrews et al., 2018; Gelb & Rutman, 2011; Marcellus, 2016; Tarasoff et al., 2018). Evidence from research to-date indicates that programs that integrate practical and social supports with prenatal and postnatal health services, such as culture, transportation, child care and meals, that address the fear of child apprehension and increase accessibility to multiple services are able to better engage women who otherwise are likely to mistrust and avoid formal systems of care (Gelb & Rutman, 2011; Marcellus, 2016; Meixner et al., 2016; Rutman & Hubberstey, 2019). Moreover, programs that use non-judgmental, relationship-based, trauma-informed and harm-reducing approaches and that acknowledge the realities of mothering have been found to be most effective in reaching pregnant women and new mothers with substance use concerns (Gelb & Rutman, 2011; Nathoo et al., 2015; Network Action Team on FASD Prevention, 2010; Pepler et al., 2014). These programs are identifying the importance of responding to the needs of women, of children and of the mother-child dyad (Tarasoff et al., 2018). Moreover, when offered with indigenous clientele or in indigenous communities, these programs increase cultural connections by integrating indigenous knowledge, worldviews and practices and by addressing intergenerational trauma and loss of culture in order to support Indigenous women's self-determination (Wolfson et al., 2019).

Despite the evidence that exists with respect to promising approaches, multi-service programs face challenges in securing adequate and continuous funding, for the diversity of programs to meet the mother's, child's and mother-child dyad's needs. At this point, few such holistic services are in place across Canada, and comparable integrated funding models are needed if they are to be sustained and expanded.

Ongoing Inaction by Health Professionals Concerning Women and Alcohol 'Brief interventions' are collaborative conversations between an individual and a health care or social service provider about alcohol use and related concerns (Nathoo et al., 2018). Brief intervention and support have been found to be an effective strategy for reducing harmful or risky alcohol use in hundreds of studies and systematic reviews (Álvarez-Bueno et al., 2015; Angus et al., 2014; Bray et al., 2011; Derges et al., 2017; Elzerbi et al., 2015; Kaner et al., 2018). National and global organizations such support the inclusion of alcohol brief interventions as a routine element of health care in all primary care settings (Center for Substance Abuse Treatment, 2009; Centers for Disease Control and Prevention, 2014; Substance Abuse and Mental Health Services Administration, 2013; World Health Organization, 2014).

Yet, a 2017 environmental scan in Canada, involving eight types of service providers in a position to discuss alcohol with girls and women of childbearing years, found that brief conversations and support about alcohol use, mental wellness, contraception and safer sex are not being routinely utilized (Nathoo et al., 2018). For service providers, a key barrier persists, which is that providers appear to fear jeopardizing their relationships with women or being perceived as judging and shaming of women's alcohol use if this topic is raised at all in clinical settings (Derges et al., 2017; Flemming et al., 2016; Johansson et al., 2005; Lock, 2004; Lynne & Peter, 2014; Muggli et al., 2015; Pilnick & Coleman, 2006; Poole et al., 2016; Stead et al., 2017). While research findings to-date indicate that the majority of women appreciate the opportunity to discuss their alcohol use and learn about ways to improve their health (Breen et al., 2014), there are numerous barriers to having open and honest discussions in clinical and community settings about alcohol use during pregnancy. Many women provide 'socially acceptable' answers or deny alcohol and substance use because they do not feel comfortable with their service provider or are concerned about involvement from the child welfare or justice systems (Boyd & Marcellus, 2007; Eichler et al., 2016; Jacobs & Jacobs, 2014; Muggli et al., 2015; Poole et al., 2016; Poole & Isaac, 2001).

We continue to need action on this basic public health strategy to ensure that all girls and women have the opportunity to engage in empowering conversations about how to reduce the harms of alcohol and, where needed, to be connected to supports.

What Does Public Health Need to Do?

The WHO's *Global strategy to reduce the harmful use of alcohol* (World Health Organization, 2010) recommends policy options and interventions available for national action in ten recommended target areas. Four of these are (a) leadership, awareness and commitment; (b) health services' response; (c) community action; and (d) monitoring and surveillance. Some examples of how this advice might be advanced in gendered ways in these four areas include:

Leadership

We need a commitment to the development of national alcohol strategies and plans for action that take sex and gender into account intersectionally. This includes 'ensuring broad access to information and effective education and public awareness programmes among all levels of society about the full range of alcohol-related harm experienced in the country and the need for, and the existence of, effective preventive measures' (p. 15).

Health Services Response

We need health and social care agencies to provide brief intervention and support on alcohol, as well as a range of harm reduction and treatment services. 'Such initiatives should include early identification and management of harmful drinking among pregnant women and women of child-bearing age' (p. 16).

Community Action

We need to support community programs and enactment of policies such as:

- Promoting municipal policies to reduce the harmful use of alcohol, including the selling of alcohol to underage drinkers and the creation of alcohol-free environments for young men and women

- Supporting community-based interventions such as the holistic services for pregnant women and new mothers and their children described in this chapter
- Supporting community programmes and policies for subpopulations at particular risks, such as young girls, lesbian and bisexual girls and indigenous girls and women

Surveillance and Monitoring

We can collect and monitor the prevalence of use, for example, by carefully capturing the prevalence of risky drinking using sex-specific measures (Poole et al., 2019) and by doing regular collection of data such as the Maternity Experiences Survey (Public Health Agency of Canada, 2009) that respectfully capture the timing and amount of drinking in pregnancy.

Action Required

Current trends in alcohol use by girls and women and heightened awareness of the factors affecting their use underscore the need to create a more gender-sensitive alcohol policy, health promotion and service delivery. We have moved at a snail's pace away from:

- Avoidance of acknowledging and addressing the harms associated with heavy drinking by girls and women in the public domain
- Inattention to policies and services that are needed to address social and structural determinants of health affecting pregnant women and new mothers and their children
- Ambivalence and inaction on the part of health and social care providers to initiate basic and informed conversations about the sex-related health effects and gender influences on alcohol use with all girls and women

Approaches that address the health and gender equity-related factors and issues on alcohol use are referred to as 'gender transformative' (Greaves et al., 2014). Gender equitable health effects will be achieved through the careful design of messaging, programming and policies so as to emphasize the power of girls and women to make health-promoting decisions and to be critical consumers of alcohol advertising. Gender-transformative approaches to alcohol will ensure that health messages are based on evidence that shows the influences of sex and gender on alcohol-related harms and tailored to specific groups of girls and women at risk of alcohol-related harms in a non-judgmental way. Gender transformative approaches will address the key influences on girls' and women's drinking and recognize the adaptive function of drinking for those in vulnerable circumstances and thus be a basis for sympathetic and empowering health promotion and service delivery that takes into account intersectional gendered issues such as violence, poverty and depression. Alcohol has been identified as a serious and urgent public health issue, and yet, its history of gender blindness and sexist practices continues to mean that this area of public health has missed numerous opportunities to be more effective and positive for girls and women. For the sake of improved health for both women and children and the prevention of FASD, we need to move past the long-standing avoidance, inattention and inaction characterizing the field. Gender-transformative approaches would empower girls and women to change harmful drinking behaviours and critique alcohol marketing. They would also promote programming and structural changes towards reducing the negative influences and factors affecting women's alcohol use. In the end, girls and women would be more aware of and educated about alcohol, more supported in making health-promoting choices, and more empowered to address and benefit from social changes that question gendered assumptions, roles and stereotypes.

References

Álvarez-Bueno, C., Rodríguez-Martín, B., García-Ortiz, L., Gómez-Marcos, M. Á., & Martínez-Vizcaíno, V. (2015). Effectiveness of brief interventions in primary health care settings to decrease alcohol consumption by adult non-dependent drinkers: A systematic review of systematic reviews. *Preventive Medicine, 76*, S33–S38. https://doi.org/10.1016/j.ypmed.2014.12.010

Andrews, N. C. Z., Motz, M., Pepler, D. J., Jeong, J. J., & Khoury, J. (2018). Engaging mothers with substance use issues and their children in early intervention: Understanding use of service and outcomes. *Child Abuse & Neglect, 83*, 10–20. https://doi.org/10.1016/j.chiabu.2018.06.011

Angus, C., Latimer, N., Preston, L., Li, J., & Purshouse, R. (2014). What are the implications for policy makers? A systematic review of the cost-effectiveness of screening and brief interventions for alcohol misuse in primary care. *Frontiers in Psychiatry, 5*, 114.

Boyd, S. C., & Marcellus, L. (2007). *With Child; Substance use during pregnancy: A woman-centred approach*. Halifax: Fernwood Publishing.

Bray, J. W., Cowell, A. J., & Hinde, J. M. (2011). A systematic review and meta-analysis of health care utilization outcomes in alcohol screening and brief intervention trials. *Medical Care, 49*(3), 287–294. https://doi.org/10.1097/MLR.0b013e318203624f

Breen, C., Awbery, E., & Burns, L. (2014). *Supporting pregnant women who use alcohol or other drugs: A review of the evidence*. Retrieved from Sydney, AU: https://ndarc.med.unsw.edu.au/resource/supporting-pregnant-women-who-use-alcohol-or-other-drugs-review-evidence

Bryans, M., Dechief, L., Hardeman, S., Marcellus, L., Nathoo, T., Poag, E., et al. (2012). *Supporting pregnant and parenting women who use substances: What communities are doing to help*. Retrieved from Vancouver, BC: http://www.canfasd.ca/files/What_Communities_Are_Doing_to_Help_February_7_2013.pdf

Caldwell, L., Schweinsburg, A., Nagel, B., Barlett, V., Brown, S., & Tapert, S. (2005). Gender and adolescent alcohol use disorders on BOLD (blood oxygen level dependent) response to spatial working memory. *Alcohol and Alcoholism, 40*(3), 194–200.

Canadian Institute for Health Information. (2017). *Alcohol harm in Canada: Examining hospitalizations entirely caused by alcohol and strategies to reduce alcohol harm*. Retrieved from Ottawa: http://www.cihi.ca/en/alcohol-harm-in-canada

Center for Substance Abuse Treatment. (2009). *Substance abuse treatment: Addressing the specific needs of women*. Retrieved from Rockville, MD.

Centers for Disease Control and Prevention. (2014). *Planning and implementing screening and brief intervention for risky alcohol use: A step-by-step guide for primary care practices.* Retrieved from Atlanta, Georgia.

Chen, W. Y., Rosner, B., Hankinson, S. E., Colditz, G. A., Willett, W. C. (2011). Moderate alcohol consumption during adult life, drinking patterns, and breast cancer risk. *JAMA., 306*(17):1884–90. https://doi.org/10.1001/jama.2011.1590. PMID: 22045766; PMCID: PMC3292347.

Cheng, H. G., Cantave, M., & Anthony, J. (2016). Taking the first full drink: Epidemiological evidence on male–female differences in the United States. *Alcoholism: Clinical and Experimental Research, 40*(4), 816–825.

Christopher I. Li, Rowan T. Chlebowski, Matthew Freiberg, Karen C. Johnson, Lewis Kuller, Dorothy Lane, Lawrence Lessin, Mary Jo O'Sullivan, Jean Wactawski-Wende, Shagufta Yasmeen, Ross Prentice. (2010). Alcohol Consumption and Risk of Postmenopausal Breast Cancer by Subtype: The Women's Health Initiative Observational Study, *JNCI: Journal of the National Cancer Institute., 102* (18):1422–31. https://doi.org/10.1093/jnci/djq316.

Chudley, A. E., Conry, J., Cook, J. L., Loock, C., Rosales, T., & LeBlanc, N. (2005). Fetal alcohol spectrum disorder: Canadian guidelines for diagnosis. *Canadian Medical Association Journal, 172*(5 suppl), S1–S21. https://doi.org/10.1503/cmaj.1040302

Crawford-Williams, F., Steen, M., Esterman, A., Fielder, A., & Mikocka-Walus, A. (2015). "My midwife said that having a glass of red wine was actually better for the baby": A focus group study of women and their partner's knowledge and experiences relating to alcohol consumption in pregnancy. *BMC Pregnancy & Childbirth, 15*(1), 1–11. https://doi.org/10.1186/s12884-015-0506-3

Derges, J., Kidger, J., Fox, F., Campbell, R., Kaner, E., & Hickman, M. (2017). Alcohol screening and brief interventions for adults and young people in health and community-based settings: A qualitative systematic literature review. *BMC Public Health, 17*, 1–12. https://doi.org/10.1186/s12889-017-4476-4

Eichler, A., Grunitz, J., Grimm, J., Walz, L., Raabe, E., Goecke, T. W., et al. (2016). Did you drink alcohol during pregnancy? Inaccuracy and discontinuity of women's self-reports: On the way to establish meconium ethyl glucuronide (EtG) as a biomarker for alcohol consumption during pregnancy. *Alcohol, 54*, 39–44. https://doi.org/10.1016/j.alcohol.2016.07.002

Elzerbi, C., Donoghue, K., & Drummond, C. (2015). A comparison of the efficacy of brief interventions to reduce hazardous and harmful alcohol consumption between European and non-European countries: A systematic review and meta-analysis of randomized controlled trials. *Addiction, 110*(7), 1082–1091. https://doi.org/10.1111/add.12960

Farhat, T., Iannotti, R., & Simons-Morton, B. (2010). Overweight, obesity, youth, and health-risk behaviors. *American Journal of Preventative Medicine, 38*(3), 258–267.

Flemming, K., Graham, H., McCaughan, D., Angus, K., Sinclair, L., & Bauld, L. (2016). Health professionals' perceptions of the barriers and facilitators to providing smoking cessation advice to women in pregnancy and during the post-partum period: A systematic review of qualitative research. *BMC Public Health, 16*(1), 1–13. https://doi.org/10.1186/s12889-016-2961-9

Gelb, K., & Rutman, D. (2011). *A literature review on promising approaches in substance use treatment and care for women with FASD.* Retrieved from Research Initiatives for Social Change Unit, University of Victoria:

Greaves, L., Pederson, A., & Poole, N. (2014). *Making it better: Gender transformative health promotion.* Toronto: Canadian Scholars Press.

Holland, C. L., Pringle, J. L., & Barbetti, V. (2009). Identification of physician barriers to the application of screening and brief intervention for problem alcohol and drug use. *Alcoholism Treatment Quarterly, 27*(2), 174–183. https://doi.org/10.1080/07347320902784890

Jacobs, L., & Jacobs, J. (2014). 'Bad' mothers have alcohol use disorder: Moral panic or brief intervention? *Gender & Behaviour, 12*(3), 5971–5979.

Jernigan, D. H., Ostroff, J., & Ross, C. (2004). Sex differences in adolescent exposure to alcohol advertising in magazines. *Archives of Pediatrics & Adolescent Medicine, 158*(7), 629–634. https://doi.org/10.1001/archpedi.158.7.629

Johansson, K., Åkerlind, I., & Bendtsen, P. (2005). Under what circumstances are nurses willing to engage in brief alcohol interventions? A qualitative study from primary care in Sweden. *Addictive Behaviors, 30*(5), 1049–1053. https://doi.org/10.1016/j.addbeh.2004.09.008

Johnston, A. D. (2011). Women are the new face of alcohol advertising. *Toronto Star.* Retrieved from http://www.thestar.com/atkinsonseries/atkinson2011/article/1090125%2D%2Dwomen-are-the-new-face-of-alcohol-advertising

Johnston, A. D. (2013). *Drink: The intiimate relationship between women and alcohol.* Toronto: Harper Collins.

Kaner, E. F. S., Beyer, F. R., Muirhead, C., Campbell, F., Pienaar, E. D., Bertholet, N., et al. (2018). Effectiveness of brief alcohol interventions in primary care populations. *Cochrane Database of Systematic Reviews, 2,* CD004148.

Kelley, M., Ehlke, S., Lewis, R., Braitman, A., Bostwick, W., Heron, K., & Lau-Barraco, C. (2018). Sexual coercion, drinking to cope motives, and alcohol-related consequences among self-identified bisexual women. *Substance Use & Misuse, 53*(7). https://doi.org/10.1080/1082608 4.2017.1400565

Kilbourne, J. (1999). *Deadly persuasion: Why women and girls must fight the addictive power of advertising.* New York: Free Press.

Kruk, E., & Banga, P. S. (2011). Engagement of substance-using pregnant women in addiction recovery. *Canadian Journal of Community Mental Health, 30*(1), 79–91.

Lock, C. A. (2004). Alcohol and brief intervention in primary health care: What do patients think? *Primary Health Care Research and Development, 5*(2), 162–178. https://doi.org/10.119 1/1463423604pc194oa

Lynne, T., & Peter, M. (2014). Smoking cessation dialogue and the complementary therapist: Reluctance to engage? *Complementary Therapies in Clinical Practice, 20*(4), 181–187. https://doi.org/10.1016/j.ctcp.2014.07.007

Marcellus, L. (2016). *Supporting families at she way and beyond.* Retrieved from Vancouver, BC: https://www.uvic.ca/hsd/nursing/assets/docs/research/faculty/lenora-sheway.pdf

Marcellus, L., MacKinnon, K., Benoit, C., Phillips, R., & Stengel, C. (2014). Reenvisioning success for programs supporting pregnant women with problematic substance use. *Qualitative Health Research, 25*(4), 500–512.

McCarty, C. A., Kosterman, R., Mason, W. A., McCauley, E., Hawkins, J. D., Herrenkohl, T. I., & Lengua, L. J. (2009). Longitudinal associations among depression, obesity and alcohol use disorders in young adulthood. *General Hospital Psychiatry, 31*(5), 442–450. https://doi.org/10.1016/j.genhosppsych.2009.05.013

Medina, K., McQueeny, T., Nagel, B., Hanson, K., Schweinsburg, A., & Tapert, S. (2008). Prefrontal cortex volumes in adolescents with alcohol use disorders: Unique gender effects. *Alcoholism: Clinical and Experimental Research, 32*(3), 386–394.

Meixner, T., Milligan, K., Urbanoski, K., & McShane, K. (2016). Conceptualizing integrated service delivery for pregnant and parenting women with addictions: Defining key factors and processes. *Canadian Journal of Addictions, 73*(3), 57–65.

Muggli, E., Cook, B., O'Leary, C., Forster, D., & Halliday, J. (2015). Increasing accurate self-report in surveys of pregnancy alcohol use. *Midwifery, 31*(3), e23–e28. https://doi.org/10.1016/j.midw.2014.11.003

Nathoo, T., Marcellus, L., Bryans, M., Clifford, D., Louie, S., Penaloza, D., et al. (2015). *Harm reduction and pregnancy: Community-based approaches to prenatal substance use in Western Canada.* Retrieved from Victoria, BC: http://bccewh.bc.ca/wp-content/uploads/2015/02/HReduction-and-Preg-Booklet.2015_web.pdf

Nathoo, T., Poole, N., Wolfson, L., Schmidt, R., Hemsing, N., & Gelb, K. (2018). *Doorways to conversation: Brief intervention on substance use with girls and women.* Retrieved from Vancouver, BC: http://bccewh.bc.ca/wp-content/uploads/2018/06/Doorways_ENGLISH_July-18-2018_online-version.pdf

Network Action Team on FASD Prevention. (2010). *10 fundamental components of FASD prevention from a women's health determinants perspective.* Retrieved from Vancouver: BC: http://www.canfasd.ca/files/PDF/ConsensusStatement.pdf

NIAAA. (2019). *Women and alcohol.* Retrieved from https://www.niaaa.nih.gov/publications/brochures-and-fact-sheets/women-and-alcohol

Niccols, A., Dell, C. A., & Clarke, S. (2010). Treatment issues for aboriginal mothers with substance use problems and their children. *International Journal of Mental Health & Addiction, 8*(2), 320–335. https://doi.org/10.1007/s11469-009-9255-8

Nolen-Hoeksema, S. (2004). Gender differences in risk factors and consequences for alcohol use and problems. *Clinical Psychology Review, 24*(8), 981–1010.

Pei, J., Kapasi, A., Kennedy, K. E., & Joly, V. (2019). *Toward healthy outcomes for individuals with FASD.* Retrieved from Edmonton, AB.

Pepler, D., Motz, M., Leslie, M., Jenkins, J., Espinet, S. D., & Reynolds, W. (2014). *A focus on relationships – The mother child study: Evaluating treatments for substance-using women.* Retrieved from http://www.mothercraft.ca/index.php?q=publications

Pilnick, A., & Coleman, T. (2006). Death, depression and 'defensive expansion': Closing down smoking as an issue for discussion in GP consultations. *Social Science & Medicine, 62*(10), 2500–2512. https://doi.org/10.1016/j.socscimed.2005.10.031

Poole, N., & Isaac, B. (2001). *Apprehensions: Barriers to treatment for substance-using mothers.* Retrieved from Vancouver, BC: http://bccewh.bc.ca/wp-content/uploads/2012/05/2001_Apprehensions-Barriers-to-Treatment-for-Substance-Using-Mothers.pdf

Poole, N., Schmidt, R. A., Bocking, A., Bergeron, J., & Fortier, I. (2019). The potential for FASD prevention of a harmonized approach to data collection about alcohol use in pregnancy. *International Journal of Environmental Research and Public Health, 16*(11). https://doi.org/10.3390/ijerph16112019

Poole, N., Schmidt, R. A., Green, C., & Hemsing, N. (2016). Prevention of Fetal alcohol Spectrum disorder: Current Canadian efforts and analysis of gaps. *Substance Abuse: Research and Treatment, 2016*(Suppl. 1), 1–11. https://doi.org/10.4137/SART.S34545

Public Health Agency of Canada. (2009). *What mothers say: The Canadian maternity experiences survey.* Retrieved from http://www.phac-aspc.gc.ca/rhs-ssg/survey-eng.php

Public Health Agency of Canada. (2018). *The chief public health officer's report on the state of public health in canada 2018: Preventing problematic substance use in youth.* Retrieved from https://www.canada.ca/en/public-health/corporate/publications/chief-public-health-officer-reports-state-public-health-canada/2018-preventing-problematic-substance-use-youth.html

Rehm, J., Taylor, B., Mohapatra, S., Irving, H., Baliunas, D., Patra, J., & Roerecke, M. (2010). Alcohol as a risk factor for liver cirrhosis: A systematic review and meta-analysis. *Drug and Alcohol Review, 29*(4), 437–445.

Rutman, D., & Hubberstey, C. (2019). National evaluation of Canadian multi-service FASD prevention programs: Interim findings from the co-creating evidence study. *International Journal of Environmental Research and Public Health, 16.* https://doi.org/10.3390/ijerph16101767

Stead, M., Parkes, T., Nicoll, A., Wilson, S., Burgess, C., Eadie, D., et al. (2017). Delivery of alcohol brief interventions in community-based youth work settings: Exploring feasibility and acceptability in a qualitative study. *BMC Public Health, 17,* 1–13. https://doi.org/10.1186/s12889-017-4256-1

Substance Abuse and Mental Health Services Administration. (2013). *Systems-level implementation of screening, brief intervention, and referral to treatment.* Retrieved from Rockville, MD.

Sword, W., Niccols, A., & Fan, A. (2004). "New Choices" for women with addictions: Perceptions of program participants. *BMC Public Health, 4,* 10–11.

Tarasoff, L., Milligan, K., Le, T., Usher, A., & Urbanoski, K. (2018). Integrated treatment programs for pregnant and parenting women with problematic substance use: Service descriptions and client perceptions of care. *Journal of Substance Abuse Treatment, 90,* 9–18. https://doi.org/10.1016/j.jsat.2018.04.008

Tuchman, E. (2010). Women and addiction: The importance of gender issues in substance abuse research. *Journal of Addictive Diseases, 29*(2), 127–138. https://doi.org/10.1080/10550881003684582

Warsh, C. K. (1993). "Oh Lord, pour a cordial in her wounded heart": The drinking woman in Victoria and Edwardian Canada. In C. K. Warsh (Ed.), *Drink in Canada, historical essays* (pp. 70–91). Montreal: McGill Queens University Press.

Watson, H., Munro, A., Wilson, M., Kerr, S., & Godwin, J. (2009). *The involvement of nurses and midwives in screening and brief interventions for hazardous and harmful use of alcohol and other psychoactive substances.* Retrieved from Geneva, Switzerland: http://apps.who.int/iris/bitstream/10665/70480/1/WHO_HRH_HPN_10.6_eng.pdf

White, A., Castle, I. J., Chen, C. M., Shirley, M., Roach, D., & Hingson, R. (2015). Converging patterns of alcohol use and related outcomes among females and males in the United States, 2002 to 2012. *Alcohol Clinical and Experimental Research, 39*(9), 1712–1726. https://doi.org/10.1111/acer.12815

Wolfson, L., Poole, N., Morton Ninomiya, M., Rutman, D., Letendre, S., Winterhoff, T., et al. (2019). Collaborative action on Fetal alcohol Spectrum disorder prevention: Principles for enacting the truth and reconciliation commission call to action #33. *International Journal of Environmental Research and Public Health, 16*(9), 1589. https://doi.org/10.3390/ijerph16091589

World Health Organization. (2010). *Global strategy to reduce the harmful use of alcohol.* Retrieved from Geneva: https://apps.who.int/iris/bitstream/handle/10665/44395/9789241599931_eng.pdf?sequence=1&isAllowed=y

World Health Organization. (2014). *Guidelines for the identification and management of substance use and substance use disorders in pregnancy.* Retrieved from Geneva, Switzerland.

Wozniak, J., Riley, E. P., & Charness, M. (2019). Clinical presentation, diagnosis, and management of fetal alcohol spectrum disorder. *Lancet Neurology, 18*(8), 760–770. https://doi.org/10.1016/S1474-4422(19)30150-4

Chapter 9
Sexual Health Promotion

Allison Carter, Karyn Fulcher, Nathan Lachowsky, and Jacqueline Gahagan

The Prevailing Framing of Sexual Health

Discourses about sexual health, in general and in public health in particular, are primarily associated with reproductive issues and STBBI prevention such as stopping negative outcomes such as HIV infection (de Visser et al., 2014; Grulich et al., 2018), unintended pregnancies (Richters et al., 2016; Taft et al., 2018), and sexual assault, harassment, and coercion (Australian Bureau of Statistics, 2017; NSW Government, 2018; Statistics Canada, 2017). Importantly, studies show enduring inequities in these sexual health outcomes between and within women, men, and gender nonbinary populations are due to a variety of social determinants, including various intersecting identities and the structural inequalities connected to them (e.g. racism, sexism, homophobia, heterosexism, trans stigma), the persistent use of the law to criminalize people and intervene in their lives and choices (e.g. sex work, drug use, migration), and other factors (e.g. unequal access to resources, heteronormative sexual scripts) that serve to inform and regulate sexuality and sexual activity

A. Carter (✉)
Kirby Institute, University of New South Wales, Sydney, NSW, Australia

Faculty of Health Sciences, Simon Fraser University, Burnaby, BC, Canada
e-mail: acarter@kirby.unsw.edu.au

K. Fulcher
School of Public Health and Social Policy, University of Victoria, Victoria, BC, Canada

N. Lachowsky
School of Public Health and Social Policy, University of Victoria, Victoria, BC, Canada

Community-Based Research Centre, Vancouver, BC, Canada

J. Gahagan
Faculty of Health, Dalhousie University, Halifax, NS, Canada

© Springer Nature Switzerland AG 2021
J. Gahagan, M. K. Bryson (eds.), *Sex- and Gender-Based Analysis in Public Health*, https://doi.org/10.1007/978-3-030-71929-6_9

(Barcelos, 2017; Bowleg et al., 2017; Burns, 2018; Krusi et al., 2012; Rosenthal & Lobel, 2018).

It is interesting to note that in Australia, there has been a 23% reduction in HIV diagnoses in 2018 compared to 2013, driven by increased prevention measures in Australian-born gay, bisexual, and men who have sex with men in major cities (e.g. regular testing, earlier treatment, strong uptake of pre-exposure prophylaxis) (Kirby Institute, 2018); this has not been witnessed in Canada at the national level. In both Australia and Canada, diagnoses in heterosexuals and Indigenous populations have been stable or increasing, particularly among Indigenous women (Kirby Institute, 2018; Public Health Agency of Canada, 2018b). In relation to sexual and/or physical violence, recently published Canadian and Australian data suggest incidents of sexual assault have remained relatively stable over the past 15 years, with the highest rates among those who are women, Indigenous, young, and gay or bisexual (NSW Government, 2018; Statistics Canada, 2017). For example, approximately one in six women and one in 16 men over the age of 15 in Australia are estimated to experience physical and/or sexual violence in their lifetime (NSW Government, 2018), a figure that is similar to countries such as the United Kingdom and the United States (Black et al., 2011).

While research on gender and social inequities in relation to negative sexual health outcomes is extremely important to advancing people's sexual safety, and well-being, affirming aspects of sexual health remain almost entirely overlooked within the current public health interventions and scientific literature (e.g. sexual agency, self-esteem, desire, pleasure, deservingness, and love) (Impett et al., 2013). A longstanding concern of feminists (Jolly et al., 2013), including those from the Global South (Bakare-Yusuf, 2013), is that risk- and deficit-focused narratives on sexuality, particularly women's sexuality, portrays marginalized populations as inherently at risk and their sexual lives as fraught with pain, disease, and suffering. This concern has also been raised by Indigenous scholars, who have advocated for a balanced approach to sexual health research and practice that values community strengths (Bell et al., 2017; Wilson et al., 2013; Yee et al., 2011). The focus on poor sexual outcomes rather than sexual pleasure or autonomy is perhaps not surprising given the focus of public health and its closely related disciplines of medicine and epidemiology, which have largely focused on the identification of disease outbreaks and control (Canadian Public Health Association, 2005). This also tends to be in line with lay definitions that equate sexual health with avoidance of sexual risk (McDaid et al., 2019). But, what would it mean to dislodge sexual health promotion approaches from the discourse on disease and medicalization and centre them on gender, pleasure, and rights in the public health narrative?

From Preventing Disease to Promoting Health: Extending Understandings of Sexual Health

The World Health Organization's initial articulation of sexual health in 1975 emphasized the positive and enhancing role that sexuality and sexual expression can have on people's lives: "Sexual health is the integration of the somatic, emotional, intellectual and social aspects of sexual being, in ways that are positively enriching and that enhance personality, communication, and love" (World Health Organization, 1975). In an effort to elaborate the concept of sexual health, Langfeldt and Porter highlighted, in 1986, another key concept: "sexuality is so much more than sexual intercourse…it is in the energy that motivates us to find love, contact, warmth, and intimacy; it is expressed in the way we feel, move, touch and are touched; it is about being sensual as well as being sexual" (p. 5) (Langfeldt & Porter, 1986). These definitions, we argue, signal the importance of a positive, holistic, and pleasure-focused view for improving people's overall sexual health, autonomy, satisfaction, and pleasure, beyond sex as a source of health-related problems.

In the ensuing decades, conceptions of sexual health and sexuality evolved further (Edwards & Coleman, 2004; Fortenberry, 2013; Robinson et al., 2002; Sandfort & Ehrhardt, 2004). One particularly important development at the turn of the millennium, emerging in response to research linking the oppressed position of women and girls to their limited access to sexual autonomy and pleasure, was recognition of the importance of sexual rights to the promotion of sexual health (Petchesky, 2000; World Association for Sexology, 1998). Sexual rights include the right of all people regardless of age, gender, race, sexual orientation, nationality, disability, socio-economic position, and so forth to have control over and make decisions concerning sex, sexuality, and sexual health, freely and without coercion, violence, or discrimination (World Association for Sexual Health, 2014; World Health Organization, 2006, p. 3). This definition recognizes the important role that sexual pleasure can play in people's lives (Abramson & Pinkerton, 2002) and advocates for comprehensive sexuality education and access to sexual health services as the foundation to sexual health promotion.

Reimagining Sexual Health through a Sex, Gender, and Social Justice Lens

Despite an overwhelming emphasis on cisgender binaries in public health, biological sex (often state-assigned at birth based on visible anatomy and physical characteristics) and gender identity (social expression that reflects how an individual sees themselves as masculine, feminine, a blend of both, neither, or something else) have several different dimensions (CIHR Institute of Gender and Health, 2018). Both sex and gender affect all aspects of sexual health and pleasure, from physiology and sexual functioning (Basson, 2000; Brotto et al., 2016; Graham, 2016); to epidemiology, health outcomes, and the social determinants of sexual health (MacPhail & McKay, 2018); to access to comprehensive sexuality education and sexual health care (Kaczkowski & Swartout, 2019); and to how bodies and sexualities are experienced and lived (Tolman et al., 2014).

Importantly, however, neither sex nor gender explanations will fully account for the differences in men's, women's, and gender-diverse people's access to and experience of sexual health outcomes and sexual pleasure, nor are they always the most important axes of identity or oppression (Crenshaw, 1989; Shields, 2008). At any time, and in every society, an individual's sex and gender and the sexual experiences across their life course that stem from these biological and social issues must be understood in relation to the intersection of a number of factors, such as race/racism, class/classism, education, income/poverty, disability, nationality, and so forth (Raphael, 2009; Wuest et al., 2002). This is because, as intersectional feminists, critical social scientists, and social epidemiologists have stressed (Collins, 1998; Crenshaw, 2000; Crenshaw et al., 2000; Hankivsky & Christoffersen, 2008; Hooks, 2000; Krieger, 2001), norms and inequalities related to sex and gender vary significantly by social position. These differences influence personal sexual experiences (e.g. behaviours, interests, and expectations) and can result in immense inequities in sexual health outcomes within (not only between) gender groups (Kaczkowski & Swartout, 2019). Thus, while sex- and gender-based analysis (SGBA) is critical to support and enhance sexual health, such approaches must be intersectional in focus and lead to interventions that aim to overcome a range of social, political, and economic hierarchies that influence sexual health outcomes (CIHR Institute of Gender and Health, 2018).

Using Sex- and Gender-Based Analysis (SGBA) to Understand and Address Sexual Health Inequities

While SGBA has been used to study a variety of sexual health topics, such as sexual agency (Closson et al., 2018), sexual desire (Graham et al., 2017), sexual satisfaction (McClelland 2010), and unplanned pregnancies (Veale et al. 2016), this is not uniformly the case, particularly in public health. The need for public health efforts to shift further upstream to advance positive approaches to sexual health that embrace people's rights to safe, satisfying, and pleasurable sex when desired—freely, consensually, and with dignity is needed. Importantly, however, much of this research does not speak to the sexual health needs and realities of gender- and socially diverse populations and remains very heterosexist and heteronormative in its focus. The importance of including the sexual and reproductive health needs and realities of populations who are often left out is in urgent need of greater focus in our sexual health efforts. This includes, but is not limited to, lesbian, gay, bisexual, trans, and queer (LGBTQ) individuals, Indigenous people, people from culturally and linguistically diverse backgrounds, people with disability, people with HIV, sex workers and people who inject drugs, and all populations that are impacted historically by marginalization. In order to deepen public health understandings and approaches to sexual health promotion, a multidisciplinary view is needed which draws from the health sciences as well as the critical social science and feminist fields, such as critical psychology, critical sociology, critical race studies, and women and gender studies.

Conclusions and Future Directions

Moving forward, several key elements of intersectionality-based SGBA in sexual health promotion are warranted in public health approaches. First and foremost, a commitment to sex- and gender-based considerations in all sexual health work is fundamental. We must consider the ways in which both sex and gender shape and are shaped by social processes, especially for populations who are pushed to the margins of society. This will require deconstructing and reconstructing new understandings of what sexual health and well-being entail in public health, not just in definition, but also in practice. There is a need to reconsider positive aspects of sexuality within sexual health promotion, if not just for the sake of sexual rights, but because these are inextricably related to health outcomes (both negative and positive). As desirable as it may seem – both politically and publicly – to remove or at least downplay the 'sexual' in 'sexual health promotion', we must ensure that our public health approach as well as our research and education convey the value and importance of positive aspects of sexuality to overall health and well-being for individuals, communities, and society at large. The era of deficits-based research and practice should be wholly rethought and shifted towards a strengths-based or resilience approach.

We have new models for sexual health promotion that include more nuanced understandings and approaches to STBBIs and sexual health more broadly. We must be mindful of the ways in which we couple or decouple sexual health from related issues of reproductive health, maternal/paternal health, and mental health. What do we lose in marrying these discourses? What opportunities do we create? Who is centred when reproduction and maternal/paternal health are incorporated? There are no universal truths to these questions but using an intersectionality-informed SGBA approach will ensure that decisions help recentre those who have been pushed to the margins of society and ameliorate persistent social and sexual inequities. The following are two examples of leadership documents from the field of sexual health that demonstrate a commitment to intersectional-based SGBA.

An excellent example is the new *Canadian Guidelines for Sexual Health Education*, which articulate core principles that align and support intersectionality informed SGBA approach to sexual health (SIECCAN, 2019). First, that comprehensive sexual health education is accessible to all people inclusive of age, race, sex, gender identity, sexual orientation, STI status, geographic location, socioeconomic status, cultural or religious background, ability, or housing status (e.g. those incarcerated, homeless, or living in care facilities). Second, that comprehensive sexual health education should promote human rights, including autonomous decision-making and respect for the rights of others. Finally, these principles articulate the need for a balanced approach that includes positive aspects of sexual and relationships with the prevention of negative outcomes. This includes having a broad-based scope and being responsive to emerging issues related to sexual health and well-being.

Another exemplar of intersectional-based SGBA work is the National Inuit Sexual Health Strategy from Pauktuutit (Pauktuutit Inuit Women of Canada, 2017). They articulated a vision of healthy Inuit sexuality that includes positive body image, healthy relationships, knowledge, pleasure and intimacy, mental wellness, self-esteem, self-determination, clear communication, consensual sex, safe sex, intergenerational communication, and LGBTQ positive. Further, they articulate the following interconnected social determinants of sexual health: housing, cost of living and food security, education, mental wellness, safety and security, intergenerational trauma, substance use, gender, health services, and stigma and discrimination.

For both examples, the critical challenge that remains is how to implement these principles and visions into the sexual health-related policies, programmes, and practices of government and non-governmental organizations. To start, we must ensure that current practitioners and frontline service providers in health care, education, and social services, as well as parents, families, and peers are provided with the resources and education necessary to raise the level of conscientiousness. In particular, public health practitioners need additional education and training on these issues in ways that are evidence-based – both in terms of content being evidence-based, but also in terms of using processes that are evidence-based and effective. This must also include the development of communication skills and professional networks that connect and bring together people with diverse lived experiences and multi-sectoral professions to collectively integrate and implement recommendations for intersectionality-based SGBA approaches to sexual health.

References

Abramson, P. R., & Pinkerton, S. D. (2002). *With pleasure: Thoughts on the nature of human sexuality*. Oxford: Oxford University Press.

Australian Bureau of Statistics. (2017). *Personal safety survey, Australia, 2016, Cat. No. 4906.0*. Retrieved from Australia: https://www.abs.gov.au/ausstats/abs@.nsf/mf/4906.0

Bakare-Yusuf, B. (2013). Thinking with pleasure: Danger, sexuality, and agency. In S. Jolly, A. Cornwall, & K. Hawkins (Eds.), *Women, sexuality and the political power of pleasure* (pp. 28–41). London: Zed Books.

Barcelos, C. (2017). Culture, contraception, and Colorblindess: Youth sexual Health promotion as a gendered racial project. *Gender & Society, 32*(2), 252–273. https://doi.org/10.1177/0891243217745314

Basson, R. (2000). The female sexual response: A different model. *Journal of Sex &Marital Therapy, 26*(1), 51–65. https://doi.org/10.1080/009262300278641

Bell, S., Aggleton, P., Ward, J., & Maher, L. (2017). Sexual agency, risk and vulnerability: A scoping review of young Indigenous Australians' sexual health. *Journal of Youth Studies, 20*(9), 1208–1224. https://doi.org/10.1080/13676261.2017.1317088

Black, M. C., Basile, K. C., Breiding, M. J., Smith, S. G., Walters, M. L., Merrick, M. T., et al. (2011). *The national intimate partner and sexual violence survey (NISVS): 2010 summary report*. Atlanta: National Center for Injury Prevention and Control, Centers for Disease Control and Prevention.

Bowleg, L., del Río-González, A. M., Holt, S. L., Pérez, C., Massie, J. S., Mandell, J. E., Boone, A., & C. (2017). Intersectional epistemologies of ignorance: How behavioral and social science research shapes what we know, think we know, and don't know about U.S. black men's sexualities. *The Journal of Sex Research, 54*(4–5), 577–603. https://doi.org/10.1080/0022449 9.2017.1295300

Brotto, L., Atallah, S., Johnson-Agbakwu, C., Rosenbaum, T., Abdo, C., Byers, E. S., et al. (2016). Psychological and interpersonal dimensions of sexual function and dysfunction. *The Journal of Sexual Medicine, 13*(4), 538–571.

Burns, M. C. (2018). Mixed messages: Inconsistent sexual scripts in Australian teenage magazines and implications for sexual health practices. *Sex Education, 18*(2), 191–205. https://doi.org/1 0.1080/14681811.2017.1415876

Canadian Public Health Association. (2005). *Public health: A conceptual framework*. Retrieved from Ottawa:

Centre for Communicable Diseases and Infection Control. (2018). A summary of the Pan-Canadian framework on sexually-transmitted and blood-borne infections. *Canadian Communicable Disease Reports, 44*(7/8), 179–181. https://doi.org/10.14745/ccdr.v44i78a05

Closson, Kalysha, Dietrich, Janan J., Lachowsky, Nathan J., Nkala, Busiwe, Palmer, Alexis, Cui, Zishan, ... Kaida, Angela. (2018). Sexual Self-Efficacy and Gender: A Review of Condom Use and Sexual Negotiation Among Young Men and Women in Sub-Saharan Africa. The Journal of Sex Research, 55(4-5), 522–539. https://doi.org/10.1080/00224499.2017.1421607.

Collins, P. H. (1998). It's all in the family: Intersections of gender, race, and nation. *Hypatia, 13*(3), 62–82.

Crenshaw, K. (1989). Demarginalizing the intersection of race and sex: A black feminist critique of antidiscrimination doctrine, feminist theory and antiracist politics. *University of Chicago Legal Forum, 1*, 139–167. http://chicagounbound.uchicago.edu/uclf/vol1989/iss1981/1988

Crenshaw, K. (2000). *Gender-related aspects of race discrimination, United Nations expert meeting on gender and racial discrimination, Zagreb, Croatia*. New York: United Nations.

Crenshaw, K., Gotanda, N., Peller, G., & Thomas, K. (2000). *Critical race theory: The key writings that formed the movement*. New York: New Press.

de Visser, R. O., Badcock, P. B., Rissel, C., Richters, J., Smith, A. M. A., Grulich, A. E., & Simpson, J. M. (2014). Safer sex and condom use: Findings from the second Australian study of Health and relationships. *Sexual Health, 11*(5), 495–504. https://doi.org/10.1071/SH14102

Edwards, W., & Coleman, E. (2004). Defining sexual health: A descriptive overview. *Archives of Sexual Behavior, 33*(3), 189–195. https://doi.org/10.1023/B:ASEB.0000026619.95734.d5

Fortenberry, J. D. (2013). The evolving sexual health paradigm: Transforming definitions into sexual health practices. *AIDS, 27*, S127–S133. https://doi.org/10.1097/QAD.0000000000000048

Graham, C. A. (2016). Reconceptualising women's sexual desire and arousal in DSM-5. *Psychology & Sexuality, 7*(1), 34–47. https://doi.org/10.1080/19419899.2015.1024469

Graham, Cynthia A., Mercer, Catherine H., Tanton, Clare, Jones, Kyle G., Johnson, Anne M., Wellings, Kaye, & Mitchell, Kirstin R. (2017). What factors are associated with reporting lacking interest in sex and how do these vary by gender? Findings from the third British national survey of sexual attitudes and lifestyles. BMJ open, 7(9), e016942-e016942. https://doi.org/10.1136/bmjopen-2017-01694.

Grulich, A. E., Guy, R., Amin, J., Jin, F., Selvey, C., Holden, J., et al. (2018). Population-level effectiveness of rapid, targeted, high-coverage roll-out of HIV pre-exposure prophylaxis in men who have sex with men: The EPIC-NSW prospective cohort study. *Lancet HIV, 5*(11), e629–e637. https://doi.org/10.1016/s2352-3018(18)30215-7

Hankivsky, O., & Christoffersen, A. (2008). Intersectionality and the determinants of health: A Canadian perspective. *Critical Public Health, 18*(3), 271–283.

Hooks, B. (2000). *Feminist theory: From margin to center*. New York: Pluto Press.

Impett, E., Muise, A., & Breines, J. (2013). From risk to pleasure: Toward a positive psychology of sexuality. In M. Hojjat & D. Cramer (Eds.), *Positive psychology of love* (pp. 57–76). New York: Oxford University Press.

Jolly, S., Cornwall, A., & Hawkins, K. (2013). *Women, sexuality and the political power of pleasure*. London: Zed Books Ltd..

Kaczkowski, W., & Swartout, K. M. (2019). Exploring gender differences in sexual and reproductive health literacy among young people from refugee backgrounds. *Culture, Health & Sexuality, 22*(4), 369–384. https://doi.org/10.1080/13691058.2019.1601772

Kirby Institute. (2018). *HIV, viral hepatitis and sexually transmissible infections in Australia: Annual surveillance report 2018.* Retrieved from Sydney: https://kirby.unsw.edu.au/report/hiv-viral-hepatitis-and-sexually-transmissible-infections-australia-annual-surveillance

Krieger, N. (2001). Theories for social epidemiology in the 21st century: An ecosocial perspective. *International Journal of Epidemiology, 30*(4), 668–677.

Krusi, A., Chettiar, J., Ridgway, A., Abbott, J., Strathdee, S. A., & Shannon, K. (2012). Negotiating safety and sexual risk reduction with clients in unsanctioned safer indoor sex work environments: A qualitative study. *American Journal of Public Health, 102*(6), 1154–1159. https://doi.org/10.2105/ajph.2011.300638

Langfeldt, T., & Porter, M. (1986). *Sexuality and family planning: Report of a consultation and research findings.* Copenhagen: World Health Organization, Regional Office for Europe.

MacPhail, C., & McKay, K. (2018). Social determinants in the sexual health of adolescent aboriginal Australians: A systematic review. *Health & Social Care in the Community, 26*(2), 131–146. https://doi.org/10.1111/hsc.12355

McClelland, Sara I. (2010). Intimate justice: A critical analysis of sexual satisfaction. Social and Personality Psychology Compass, 4(9), 663–680. https://doi.org/10.1111/j.1751-9004.2010.00293.x

McDaid, L., Hunt, K., McMillan, L., Russell, S., Milne, D., Ilett, R., & Lorimer, K. (2019). Absence of holistic sexual health understandings among men and women in deprived areas of Scotland: qualitative study. *BMC Public Health, 19*(1), 299. https://doi.org/10.1186/s12889-019-6558-y

NSW Government. (2018). *NSW sexual assault strategy 2018–2021.* Retrieved from Sydney: https://www.women.nsw.gov.au/strategies-and-resources/sexual-assault/nsw-sexual-assault-strategy

Pauktuutit Inuit Women of Canada. (2017). *National Inuit sexual health strategy.* Retrieved from Toronto: https://www.pauktuutit.ca/wp-content/uploads/Tavva_SexualHealth_English.pdf

Petchesky, R. (2000). Sexual rights: Inventing a concept, mapping an international practice. In R. M. B. R. Parker & P. Aggleton (Eds.), *Framing the sexual subject: The politics of gender, sexuality and power* (pp. 81–103). Berkeley: University of California Press.

Public Health Agency of Canada. (2018b). *Summary: Estimates of HIV incidence, prevalence and Canada's progress on meeting the 90-90-90 HIV targets, 2016.* Retrieved from Ottawa: https://www.canada.ca/en/public-health/services/publications/diseases-conditions/summary-estimates-hiv-incidence-prevalence-canadas-progress-90-90-90.html

Raphael, D. (2009). *Social determinants of health: Canadian perspectives* (2nd ed.). Toronto: Canadian Scholars' Press.

Richters, J., Fitzadam, S., Yeung, A., Caruana, T., Rissel, C., Simpson, J. M., & de Visser, R. O. (2016). Contraceptive practices among women: The second Australian study of health and relationships. *Contraception, 94*(5), 548–555. https://doi.org/10.1016/j.contraception.2016.06.016

Robinson, B. B. E., Bockting, W. O., Simon Rosser, B. R., Miner, M., & Coleman, E. (2002). The Sexual Health model: Application of a sexological approach to HIV prevention. *Health Education Research, 17*(1), 43–57. https://doi.org/10.1093/her/17.1.43

Rosenthal, L., & Lobel, M. (2018). Gendered racism and the sexual and reproductive health of Black and Latina women. *Ethnicity & Health, 25*(3), 367–392. https://doi.org/10.1080/13557858.2018.1439896

Sandfort, T. G., & Ehrhardt, A. A. (2004). Sexual health: A useful public health paradigm or a moral imperative? *Archives of Sexual Behavior, 33*(3), 181–187. https://doi.org/10.1023/B:ASEB.0000026618.16408.e0

Shields, S. A. (2008). Gender: An intersectionality perspective. *Sex Roles, 59*(5), 301–311. https://doi.org/10.1007/s11199-008-9501-8

SIECCAN. (2019). *2019 Canadian guidelines for sexual health education.* Retrieved from Toronto: http://sieccan.org/sexual-health-education/

Statistics Canada. (2017). *Self-reported sexual assault in Canada, 2014.* Ottawa: Statistics Canada.

Taft, A. J., Shankar, M., Black, K. I., Mazza, D., Hussainy, S., & Lucke, J. C. (2018). Unintended and unwanted pregnancy in Australia: a cross-sectional, national random telephone survey of prevalence and outcomes. *Medical Journal of Australia, 209*, 407–408.

Tolman, D. L., Bowman, C. P., & Fahs, B. (2014). Sexuality and embodiment. In L. M. Diamond (Ed.), *APA handbook of sexuality and psychology* (Vol. 1, pp. 759–804). Person-Based Approaches.

Veale, Jaimie, Watson, Ryan, Adjei, Jones, & Saewyc, Elizabeth. (2016). Prevalence of Pregnancy Involvement Among Canadian Transgender Youth and its Relation to Mental Health, Sexual Health, and Gender Identity. International Journal of Transgenderism, 17, 1–7. https://doi.org/1 0.1080/15532739.2016.1216345.

Wilson, D., de la Ronde, S., Brascoupé, S., Apale, A. N., Barney, L., Guthrie, B., et al. (2013). Health professionals working with first nations, Inuit, and Métis consensus guideline: Chapter 5 first nations, Inuit, and Métis women's sexual and reproductive health. *Journal of Obstetrics and Gynaecology Canada, 35*(6), S28–S32. https://doi.org/10.1016/S1701-2163(15)30705-2

World Association for Sexology. (1998). Valencia declaration on sexual rights. *Scandinavian Journal of Sexology, 1*(80).

World Association for Sexual Health. (2014). *Declaration of sexual rights*. Retrieved from http://www.worldsexology.org

World Health Organization. (1975). *Education and treatment in human sexuality: The training of health professionals (Technical Report Series No. 572)*. Retrieved from Geneva:

World Health Organization. (2006). *Defining sexual health: Report of a technical consultation on sexual health*. Geneva: World Health Organization.

Wuest, J., Merritt-Gray, M., Berman, H., & Ford-Gilboe, M. (2002). Illuminating social determinants of Women's Health using grounded theory. *Health Care for Women International, 23*, 794–808.

Yee, J., Apale, A. N., Deleary, M., & Wilson, D. (2011). Sexual and reproductive health, rights, and realities and access to services for first nations, Inuit, and Métis in Canada. *Journal of Obstetrics and Gynaecology Canada, 33*(6), 633–637. https://doi.org/10.1016/S1701-2163(16)34914-3

Chapter 10
Understanding Pandemics Through a Sex- and Gender-Based Analysis Plus (SGBA+) Lens

Olena Hankivsky

During pandemics, existing inequities are exacerbated, increasing vulnerabilities to disease among those who are socially, economically, and geographically disadvantaged and who already experience a disproportionate burden of poor health. Both individuals and populations have different susceptibility to disease if they are exposed, different levels of exposures when pandemics strike, and differential access to timely and appropriate treatments (e.g. Crooks et al., 2018; Doyal, 2013; Pirtle, 2020). Research evidence also demonstrates significant differences in how regions and countries around the world experience pandemics due to geographic location, public health emergency preparedness measures, strengths of existing healthcare systems, and resources available to respond to such emergencies (Lebeaux, 2016; McLafferty, 2010; San Martin et al., 2019). There is a growing body of knowledge on the specific factors and contexts indicating the magnitude of the disproportionate impacts on the poor, disadvantaged, and socially marginalized populations. For example, the gendered impacts of pandemics have been increasingly highlighted, resulting in calls to action to respond to these effects (e.g. Patton, 2005; Purdie et al., 2020; Richardson et al., 2014; Smith, 2019, 2020; Wenham et al., 2020).

To date, however, understandings of the differential impacts of pandemics on men, women, boys, and girls of diverse backgrounds have been hampered by the relative lack of attention to the interplay of complex factors and influencing forces that underpin pandemics, including but not limited to, gender. Specifically, what is needed is a more sophisticated and transformative analysis. The purpose of this chapter is to explore the potential of sex- and gender-based analysis plus (SGBA+) to advance such an analysis (see Chap. 12 for the full treatment of SGBA+ in relation to gender-transformative approaches). Specific calls have recently been made

O. Hankivsky (✉)
Centre for Health Equity, Melbourne School of Population and Global Health, University of Melbourne, Carlton, VIC, Australia
e-mail: o.hankivsky@unimelb.edu.au

© Springer Nature Switzerland AG 2021
J. Gahagan, M. K. Bryson (eds.), *Sex- and Gender-Based Analysis in Public Health*, https://doi.org/10.1007/978-3-030-71929-6_10

in Canada, for example, for the country as a whole to deepen its commitment to SGBA+ in research and policy in the current COVID-19 era (Bauer, 2020).

The focus of this chapter is to examine what this would entail and, in particular, to interrogate the + in this tool – intersectionality. I discuss what intersectionality requires of SGBA+ and the implications for worldwide public health crises that have threatened the global community such as severe acute respiratory syndrome (SARS), Ebola, Zika, and most recently COVID-19. Through an examination of these examples, I illustrate what has been emphasized and what is often missing in the analysis of public health emergencies and pandemics. I also demonstrate the value added of an intersectionality multi-level power-focused analysis of interacting factors, processes, and structures for generating better evidence to advance understandings and responses to pandemics.

Recent Public Health Emergencies

Severe Acute Respiratory Syndrome (SARS)

Severe acute respiratory syndrome (herein, SARS) was first reported in Asia in February of 2003 (CDC, 2004). SARS is a viral respiratory disease caused by a strain of coronavirus (CDC, 2004). The virus is spread through close contact with an infected individual through coughing or sneezing, or through contact with contaminated surfaces (CDC, 2004). The virus results in a high fever, other flu-like symptoms, and most patients develop pneumonia as a result. By the end of the pandemic, 8098 people were infected globally across two dozen countries in North America, South America, and Europe. This resulted in 774 deaths (CDC, 2004, p. 1).

In examining the spread of, in this case, SARS, a number of contributing factors have been identified in the literature starting with the fact that more than 30% of the global population lives in East and Southeast Asia, which is an area of significant known pools of human pathogens (Horby et al., 2013). The region is host to a large and diverse population of mammalian wildlife species and domestic livestock, acting as reservoirs or amplifying species from which new infectious diseases of humans might emerge. Urbanization, poverty, and internal migration between rural and urban settings and thereby transferring pathogens from rural ecosystems have also been identified as contributing public health problems (Horby et al., 2013).

Public health surveillance and slow public health responses, especially in China, where the outbreak started, were especially salient. Not only was it the case that few countries possessed the necessary surveillance and response capacities to rapidly detect and control emerging infectious diseases, but also there were specific issues with respect to SARS in terms of underreporting. According to Heymann (2013), the outbreak occurred at a time when many countries hesitated reporting infectious disease outbreaks to the World Health Organization (WHO), in large part because they feared damage to national economies.

Travel, and specifically the travel of one patient from Hong Kong to Canada, was also cited as contributing to the spread of SARS (Braden et al., 2013). In analysing the experience of SARS in Toronto, the hardest hit location after China and Hong Kong, the Government of Canada noted that the outbreak placed unprecedented demands on the public health system and that Canada, with its relatively robust healthcare system, was not in fact ready to deal with the implications associated with a full-blown pandemic (Pubic Health Agency of Canada, 2003).

The erosion of public healthcare systems through privatization and weakening disease surveillance systems have been attributed as key reasons for differential outcomes related to the SARS pandemic (Farmer, 2003). Gendered effects were also documented with males being more severely affected than females (Karlberg et al., 2004), and SARS was shown to be more severe during pregnancy than at other times (Anker, 2007; Jamieson et al., 2006). In Canada, for example, nurses (who were predominantly female) reported greater negative impacts in terms of stress than medical doctors who were primarily male (Maunder, 2004), leading to calls to incorporate gender issues into public health infectious disease outbreak management programmes to improve the continuum of care throughout all phases (prevention, preparedness, and response) (Amaratunga et al., 2010).

Ebola

Late in December of 2013, the first case of Ebola was found in what would become the 2014 West African Ebola outbreak. The virus, which typically affects people living in or near tropical rainforests, is most commonly transmitted between humans via sweat, blood, secretions, or other bodily fluids or organs. The virus progresses through different stages – beginning with fever and escalating to vomiting, diarrhoea, internal and external bleeding followed by death. The most recent outbreak of Ebola began in a small village in Guinea and spread throughout the country, as well as to Sierra Leone and Liberia (CDC, 2016a; WHO, 2015a). That same year, the WHO confirmed Ebola as a 'public health emergency of international concern' (WHO, 2014). As of April 2016, in the three aforementioned countries, there had been a total of 28,616 cases (including suspected, probable, and confirmed cases) of which 15,227 were lab-confirmed cases, resulting in 11,310 deaths (CDC, 2019a). While the 2014–2016 outbreak was considered the largest and most complex, Ebola outbreaks continue with the most recent case being reported in May 2020 in the Democratic Republic of the Congo (CDC, 2020).

High levels of deforestation in Guinea have increasingly brought wild animals into contact with human populations, including bats that are theorized to be a reservoir for the disease (WHO, 2015a). As will be described, the WHO notes that unlike equatorial Africa, which had experience with outbreaks of Ebola, West African public health systems were unprepared for Ebola (WHO, 2015b). The transmission within communities, and its appearance in major urban centres (including each of the capitals of the three affected nations), were significant factors in the spread of Ebola (WHO, 2015b).

As has been noted elsewhere (Hankivsky, 2015), this public health crisis has been framed in a myriad of ways. The socioeconomic position and the history of regional instability are considered to have played a major part in contributing to the disease's spread (WHO, 2015b). Worsening socioeconomic conditions also precipitate cross-border movements of people between the highly porous borders of nations in affected regions in search of money and food, increasing the risk of transmission (WHO, 2015b). At the same time, the closure of borders and travel restrictions often hindered access to markets for cross-border and daily market traders, the majority of whom are women. Both women who continued to travel to earn money, as well as women who had to work less to care for the sick at home, were at increased risk of acquiring the infection (Fawole et al., 2016). Other evidence points to the importance of hunting – a predominant livelihood for men – as a catalyst of the outbreak (Nkangu et al., 2017). Lastly, a lack of healthcare workers and safe work conditions also contributed to the spread (WHO, 2015b).

Geography has also been offered as a key reason for the slow international response, including that of the WHO, and the inadequate healthcare system. This is most starkly evidenced by the fact that the development of drugs and vaccines is not prioritized for diseases that affect poor and remote countries. There is no doubt the reaction of the pharmaceutical industry would have been very different if the outbreak had occurred in some large Western nation (Hankivsky, 2015). Experimental drugs such as ZMapp seem to be more readily available to patients from the West. This was evidenced by the death of a leading Ebola doctor in Sierra Leone who did not receive ZMapp, while two re-patriated American aid workers did and survived.

Others have raised the issue of race and racism. In the United States, critics have argued that Thomas Eric Duncan died in Dallas because the "white man" withheld medical treatment to him (Kim & Jackson, 2014). Similarly, the Giorgis (2014) article, "The problem with the west's Ebola response is still fear of a black patient," suggested that Ebola was being framed as a "black" disease, in a way that perpetuates racism. Dionne and Seay (2015) have similarly noted that the Ebola outbreak highlights ethnocentric and xenophobic understandings of Africa, including the myths and stereotypes of Africans and the African continent as diseases and monolithic geographic setting.

Others yet have argued that gender played a key role (Davies & Bennett, 2016; Harman, 2016; UN Women IASC, 2015). Indeed, it is estimated that as many as 75% of Ebola deaths in Liberia were among females, no doubt largely due to the gendered division of informal and formal care work, including frontline care of sick patients and relatives (UN Women, 2014). Women also traditionally prepare bodies for burial, which placed them at particular risk of exposure to Ebola (Davies & Bennett, 2016). And yet, there have been serious critiques about the lack of attention to gender and specifically women within the analysis of and international response to the Ebola outbreak. Harman (2016) enumerates these as conspicuous invisibility of women and gender in available data, narratives on Ebola, emergency and long-term strategies to contain the disease, academic debates on the response, and the health system strengthening plans of the WHO and World Bank.

And finally, religion and spirituality, with promises of traditional healings, have been noted as key reasons for undermining uptake of public health measures such as treatment and care of those with the virus. Cultural mourning practices were attributed to a considerable number of infections. For example, information produced in August 2014 by the Guinean Ministry of Health suggested that 60% of cases could be linked back to burial rites, and in November 2014 WHO staff estimated the link to have caused 80% of cases in Sierra Leone (WHO, 2015b).

Zika

Zika is a mosquito-borne virus first identified in humans in Uganda and the United Republic of Tanzania in 1952. Brazil was the starting place for the latest major outbreak of the disease in 2015. Although mosquitoes are the primary vector of infection, the virus has been linked to sexual transmission as well (CDC, 2019b). While Zika fever is quite mild, requiring no hospitalization for the vast majority of those infected, the disease has been linked to microcephaly in infants born to women infected during pregnancy and Guillain-Barré syndrome (WHO, 2016a).

An analysis of Zika has been linked to environmental factors, including climate variations, urbanization, land use change, and deforestation. A recent review of the virus suggests that such factors have contributed to "a new regime" of virus transmission (Ali et al., 2017, p. 1). In particular, deforestation and climate change serve to increase favourable conditions for the breeding of mosquitoes and for positively accelerating the mosquitoes' life cycle (Ali et al., 2017; WHO, 2016b).

Poverty has also been a recognized factor in the spread and impact of Zika. As part of the WHO's travel advice preceding the 2016 Summer Olympic games held in Rio, Brazil, the organization suggested that travellers avoid visiting impoverished and overcrowded areas in cities and towns with no piped water and poor sanitation (ideal breeding grounds of mosquitoes), where the risk of being bitten is higher (WHO, 2016c).

In addition, during the initial outbreak of Zika, links between the location of microcephaly cases, poverty, public health, the women most affected—the urban poor, the Indigenous in remote locations—and their lack of access to contraceptives and abortion emerged as gender-based matters of particular concern (Davies & Bennett, 2016; Fried & Liebowitz, 2016; Fried & Welbourn, 2016; Schmidt, 2016). In general, the combination of poverty, marginalised communities, deteriorating infrastructure, and lack of piped water has been noted by several sources as contributing to the spread of mosquito-borne illnesses and, in turn, the spread of Zika as well (Basu, 2016; Vittor, 2016; Watts, 2016). To illustrate, Zika has been positioned as an epidemic that overwhelmingly affects poor black and brown women in under-resourced parts of Brazil, and as such underscores inequalities related to race, poverty and gender (Stern, 2016).

COVID-19

The COVID-19 pandemic is considered as the most crucial global public health crisis of the century, the greatest challenge that humankind has faced since the Second World War, and a pandemic of unprecedented social and economic impacts (Chakraborty & Maity, 2020). In December 2019, a new infectious respiratory disease emerged in Wuhan, Hubei province, China and was named by the WHO as COVID-19 (coronavirus disease 2019). To date over 200 countries worldwide have been affected and over 20 million cases have been reported as well as over 750,000 deaths (Johns Hopkins, 2020).

While much attention is focused on developing a safe vaccine and effective therapeutics against COVID-19, greater attention is also being paid to the health, economic, social and environmental effects of the pandemic across populations. Concerns have been raised over the disproportionate risks and impacts on the elderly, on migrant and refugee populations, on persons with disabilities, and on racial and ethnic minority populations (Bowleg, 2020; Lee & Miller, 2020). For example, in Toronto, Canada 83% of cases between May and July 2020 were among racialized populations. Another study using data from April 2020 found that nearly 20% of U.S. counties that are disproportionately black accounted for 52% of COVID-19 diagnoses and 58% of COVID-19 deaths nationally (Millett et al., 2020). Other research has shown COVID-19's disproportionate impact on migrants; as of mid-June 2020, migrants accounted for at least 8% of the population in 8 of the 15 countries with the highest number of COVID-19 cases (IOM GMDAC, 2020). This share was more than 13% in four of these countries (ibid.), a reflection of their overrepresentation given that the global share of international migrants make up 3.5% of the total population (Johnstone & Momani, 2020; Migration Data Portal, 2020). Calls have also been made internationally for explicit attention to the gendered impacts of COVID-19 given that while severity of illness and morbidity are higher in men, women have been reported to experience more vulnerabilities vis-a-vis COVID-19 because they are the majority of frontline health and care workers, and bear a greater burden of domestic violence, household and childcare responsibilities, mental health, and economic impacts of the pandemic (Wenham et al., 2020).

Looking at Pandemics with a New Lens

Reactions to the public health emergencies related to pandemics have generally focused on finding solutions to containing viruses and generating insights intended to ensure learning important lessons, especially in terms of strengthening healthcare systems and developing effective interventions for the future. And while single explanatory factors have been noted, such as geography, race/ethnicity, religion, gender, and socioeconomic status, and other pandemic determinants have received comparatively less attention, with the exception of Zika and arguably more recently with COVID-19, little attention has been paid to *explicitly* interrogating the complex interplay of factors underpinning pandemics from an intersectional perspective.

As COVID-19, in particular, has shown, people have differential exposure to and risk for the virus, different access to timely and appropriate treatment and different mortality outcomes. As is now well understood, COVID-19 has exacerbated and amplified existing social and health inequities, including gender inequality, not only between groups but within them as well (CHRC, 2020; FAO, 2020; Preworski, 2020). Even before this current pandemic Nunes (2016) argued that alternative framings of pandemics are needed that explicitly consider power inequalities, relations between groups and the production of harm, vulnerability and structural violence that result from such processes and supporting structures. For example, in the current era of COVID-19, this means moving from generalised population-based mitigation strategies to focusing on those most at risk of severe outcomes from COVID-19, including in relation to policies that are put into place to mitigate and respond to the pandemic (Schwalbe et al., 2020). For the 'pandemic era in which we live' (Morens et al., 2009) a more sophisticated and intersectional approach is urgently required.

Understanding the '+' in SGBA+ analysis of Pandemics

The '+' in SGBA+ has potential for assisting in such alternative framings as it explicitly highlights intersectionality, which has been recognized as an effective approach for capturing multiple and interactive factors, structures and processes of power. This potential has been recognized by others who have examined GBA+ (on which SGBA+ is modelled) in the Canadian context. For example, Johnstone and Momani (2020) argue, "Only with an intersectional lens on the impact of COVID-19 on society will we see the differentiated impact of this virus on individuals and communities". Further, calls for action to the Canadian government have been made by women's advocacy groups to ensure the application of an intersectionality lens to COVID-19 (Canadian Women's Foundation, 2020; Wright, 2020).

From an intersectionality perspective (see Chap. 13 for a full exploration), the dynamics of pandemics cannot be reduced to simple foci or list of explanatory factors (or necessarily ranking of factors of importance) whose influence is measured by summing up their cumulative effects. What is required, is explicit attention to their *intersecting* – that is, the dynamic relationship, where each shapes and influences each another in creating a disease experience and outcome for affected populations. At the same time, as Rita Dhamoon (2011) highlights, an intersectionality type of analysis is not just focused on actual intersections but instead interrogates what they reveal about systems of power: specifically, multilevel, interacting systems and structures at the global context, in which individual experiences are embedded. Structural inequalities created by these interacting systems and structures, across time and place, are essential to recognize and interrogate pandemics.

There is important foundational being developed in this regard. For example, in their examination of Zika and Ebola, Davies and Bennett (2016), attempt to position their analysis as advancing more nuanced understandings of gendered dimensions. They argue, for example, that:

> … in writing about gender we recognize and acknowledge the multiplicity of cross-cutting factors that characterize women's lives. Accordingly, in analyzing gender we also acknowledge the interdependence of age, disability, race, ethnicity, sexuality and socio-economic status in shaping the lived experience and health outcomes of women and girls, as well as men and boys (Davies & Bennett, 2016, p. 1044).

Nevertheless, this acknowledgement does not translate into a defining feature of their analysis but conversely, as noted throughout their article, it highlights the disproportionate effects on certain women with fewer resources in low- and middle-income countries. Primacy and dominant attention are still given to a static notion of a gender binary throughout the analysis.

With COVID-19, significant attention has been paid to the gendered and disproportionate effects on women and girls, and powerful arguments have been made that public health responses to pandemics that do not incorporate gender analysis serve to further exacerbate inequities (Smith, 2020).

And yet, as Hankivsky and Kapilashrami (2020) point out:

> …simply prioritising women and building in a sex-and-gender focus won't paint the full picture of COVID-19's impact or provide us with enough information in order to fully address it. When only impacts on 'women' or 'men' are considered, there is a risk of homogenizing otherwise diverse experiences and reducing analysis to the simplistic messaging that 'pandemics affect women and men differently.' A narrow gender focus can reinforce binary and competing understandings of the burden posed by COVID-19 on women versus men (Hankivsky & Kapilashrami, 2020)

In comparison, an application of intersectionality would not result in any predetermined hierarchy of vulnerable groups or universal conception of their experiences. Rather, intersectionality-informed analyses demonstrate that risks and impacts are shaped by a *web of intersecting factors,* which cannot be reduced to sex and gender but include sex, gender, age, health status, geographic location, disability, migration status, race/ethnicity, and socioeconomic status. Further, intersectionality examines how factors experienced at individual and group levels are shaped by broader processes and structures of power to create an interplay of advantages and vulnerabilities (Hankivsky & Kapilashrami, 2020). This offers a critical conceptional and practical rethinking of public health responses that can help resist against static framing of inequality and disadvantage in the face of pandemics.

Intersectionality can thus lead to better capturing experiences of different groups of women, men and gender-diverse people and recognizing gender as an intersecting component of wider structural inequalities. For example, as noted previously (Hankivsky, 2015), an intersectionality-informed public health analysis would interpret factors, such as geography (including urban/rural location), race, gender, and socioeconomic status, that operate together in a synergistic fashion to shape the experiences of those affected by pandemic crises. To illustrate, a "female Ebola patient" is not only defined by gender but also by her interacting geographic location, race, socioeconomic status, and religion (Hankivsky, 2015). It may also be the case that within these interactions, gender may not figure as prominently as other contributing factors. Recently, the Gender and Health Unit at Health Canada in its guide *COVID-19 and Sex, Gender and Intersectionality* similarly acknowledged, "We know that health risks, burdens, experiences and outcomes are different for everyone. In responses to COVID-19, we need to consider intersecting factors such as age, geography, disability, race/ethnicity and Indigeneity, migration/refugee status, class, and other structural conditions, including precarious housing, employment, and political and environmental stressors" (Health Canada, 2020).

For the '+' in SGBA+ to be accurately implemented, a number of important changes would need to be made. First, capacity and expertise among health researchers and public health decision-makers would need to increase in terms of understanding and operationalizing intersectionality (e.g. Hankivsky & Mussell, 2019) and better understanding the types of data needed (and from which sources) in order to be able to undertake an intersectionality-informed analysis. Data that are disaggregated only by sex, gender or age, for example, are not robust enough for such an intersectional analysis. Disaggregating outbreak-related data with an intersectional lens has been recognized as crucial in helping guide the international community's prevention and response efforts (e.g. Cleveland, 2020). Priority would also need to be given to a combination of research methods – qualitative, quantitative and mixed methods – to ensure that the lived experience of those most affected is accurately captured.

Public health policy-makers would need to resist an a priori ranking of factors or population groups in pandemic planning and responses, and even when fine-grained analysis of disproportionate risks and effects are noted, attention should be paid to individual and community-based resilience in the face of pandemics. Intersectoral collaborations and actions would need to increase to ensure that sectors shaping health beyond health systems such as education, social protection, housing, labour and law are accounted for. Beyond the national levels, public health decision-makers would need to zoom out and account for the broader structures of power internationally and globally that interact to shape the conditions for outbreaks and spread of pandemics – the 'causes of the causes' such as globalization, capitalism, urbanization, war, conflict, climate change, racism and xenophobia. As Bowleg so persuasively argues, "Now, and when COVID-19 ends, we—policymakers, public health officials, and all of us who care about public health—have a moral imperative to centre and equitably address the health, economic, and social needs of those who bear the intersectional brunt of structural inequality" (Bowleg, 2020, p. 917).

Conclusion

At a minimum, public health solutions to future pandemics may lie in strengthening healthcare systems that are, at present, weak and in creating effective processes for developing drugs and vaccines for rare diseases. But these measures in and of themselves will not sufficiently buffer against future pandemics or inform how current public healthcare responses can address the ongoing challenges of COVID-19 and future outbreaks across different countries and populations. As this chapter has discussed, new public health approaches are urgently needed to better understand and mitigate the impacts of pandemics. In this way the SGBA+ approach, with its explicit attention to the integration of intersectionality, holds much promise. Intersectionality reveals the complex interplay of risks and effects of pandemics at multiple levels and provides important insights into what needs to transpire for transformation of power to not only deal with the current COVID-19 crisis but also with future pandemics that threaten the entire international community.

References

Ali, S., Gugliemini, O., Harber, S., Harrison, A., Houle, L., Ivory, J., et al. (2017). Environmental and social change drive the explosive emergence of Zika virus in the Americas. *PLoS Neglected Tropical Diseases, 11*(2), e0005135.

Amaratunga, C., Phillips, K. P., O'Connor, E., O'Sullivan, T. L., Boscoe, M., Lemyre, L., & Krewski, D. (2010). *The need for healthcare worker sex and gender-sensitive supports during infectious disease outbreaks. SARS unmasked: Risk communication of pandemics and influenza in Canada* (pp. 172–187). Montreal: McGill-Queen's University Press.

Anker, M. (2007). Pregnancy and emerging diseases. *Emerging Infectious Diseases, 13*(3), 518–519.

Basu, A. (2016). *Zika, poverty, and reproductive health.* United Nations Foundation. January 29, 2016. http://unfoundationblog.org/zika-poverty-and-reproductive-health/. Accessed 2 Aug 2020

Bauer, G. (2020). Why Canada needs to deepen its commitment to SGBA+ in research and policy. *The Hill Times.* 1726: 28.

Bowleg, L. (2020). We're not all in this together: On COVID-19, intersectionality, and structural inequality. *American Journal of Public Health, 110*, 917.

Braden, C. R., Dowell, S. F., Jernigan, D. B., & Hughes, J. M. (2013). Progress in global surveillance and response capacity 10 years after severe acute respiratory syndrome. *Emerging Infectious Diseases, 19*(6), 864.

Canadian Human Rights Commission. (2020). *Statement – Inequality amplified by COVID-19 crisis.* https://www.chrc-ccdp.gc.ca/eng/content/statement-inequality-amplified-covid-19-crisis. Accessed 3 Aug 2020.

Canadian Women's Foundation. (2020). *Advocating for a strong gender lens on the COVID-19 Pandemic.* https://canadianwomen.org/blog/gender-lens-on-covid-19/. Accessed 1 Aug 2020

CDC. (2004). *Fact sheet: Basic information about SARS.* http://www.cdc.gov/sars/about/fs-sars.pdf. Accessed 3 Aug 2020

CDC. (2016a). https://www.cdc.gov/vhf/ebola/outbreaks/drc/2020-june.html

CDC. (2019a). *2014–2016 Ebola outbreak in West Africa.* https://www.cdc.gov/vhf/ebola/history/2014-2016-outbreak/index.html. Accessed 20 Jul 2020

CDC. (2019b). *Zika virus: Sexual transmission and prevention.* https://www.cdc.gov/zika/prevention/sexual-transmission-prevention.html. Accessed 18 Aug 2020

CDC. (2020). *Democratic Republic of the Congo, Equateur province (ongoing).* https://www.cdc.gov/vhf/ebola/outbreaks/drc/2020-june.html. Accessed 2 Aug 2020

Chakraborty, I., & Maity, P. (2020). COVID-19 outbreak: Migration, effects on society, global environment and prevention. *Science of the Total Environment, 723*, 138882.

Cleveland, N. (2020). *An intersectional approach to a pandemic? Gender data, disaggregation, and COVID-19.* https://data2x.org/an-intersectional-approach-to-a-pandemic-gender-data-disaggregation-and-covid-19/. Accessed 15 Jun 2020.

Crooks, K., Massey, P. D., Taylor, K., Miller, A., Campbell, S., & Andrews, R. (2018). Planning for and responding to pandemic influenza emergencies: it's time to listen to, prioritize and privilege Aboriginal perspectives. *Western Pacific Surveillance and Response Journal, 9*(5 Suppl 1), 5.

Davies, S. E., & Bennett, B. (2016). A gendered human rights analysis of Ebola and Zika: Locating gender in global health emergencies. *International Affairs, 92*(5), 1041–1060.

Dhamoon, R. K. (2011). Considerations on mainstreaming intersectionality. *Political Research Quarterly, 64*(1), 230–243.

Dionne, K. Y., & Seay, L. (2015). Perceptions about Ebola in America: Othering and the role of knowledge about Africa. *Political Science & Politics, 48*, 6–7.

Doyal, L. (2013). *Living with HIV and dying with AIDS: Diversity, inequality, and human rights in the global pandemic.* London: Taylor & Francis.

Farmer, P. (2003). SARS and inequality. *The nation* Accessed on https://www.thenation.com/article/sars-and-inequality/. Accessed 20 Nov 2016

Fawole, O. I., Bamiselu OF, Adewuyi, P. A., & Nguku, P. M. (2016). Gender dimensions to the Ebola outbreak in Nigeria. *Annals of African Medicine, 15*(1), 7–13.

Food and Agriculture Organization of the United Nations. (2020). *Addressing inequality in times of COVID-19.* https://reliefweb.int/sites/reliefweb.int/files/resources/CA8843EN.pdf. Accessed 30 Jul 2020.

Fried, S. T., & Liebowitz, D. J. (2016). What the solution isn't: The parallel of the Zika and HIV viruses for women. *Lancet Global Health.* https://marlin-prod.literatumonline.com/pb-assets/Lancet/langlo/TLGH_Blogs_2013-2018.pdf. Accessed 2 Aug 2020.

Fried, S. T., & Welbourn, A. (2016). *The confinement of eve: resolving Ebola, Zika and HIV with women's bodies?* Open Democracy https://www.opendemocracy.net/en/5050/confinement-of-eve-resolving-ebola-zika-and-hiv-with-women-s-bodi/. Accessed 25 Jul 2020

Giorgis, H. (2014). The problem with the west's ebola response is still fear of a black patient. *The Guardian.* https://www.theguardian.com/commentisfree/2014/oct/16/west-ebola-response-black-patient. Accessed 2 Jun 2015

Hankivsky, O. (2015). Intersectionality and Ebola. *Political Science and Politics, 48*(1), 14–15.

Hankivsky, O., & Kapilashrami, A. (2020). Intersectionality offers a radical rethinking of COVID-19. *The BMJ Opinion.* https://blogs.bmj.com/bmj/2020/05/15/intersectionality-offers-a-radical-rethinking-of-covid-19/. Accessed 15 Jul 2020

Hankivsky, O., & Mussell, L. (2019). Gender-based analysis plus in Canada: Problems and possibilities of integrating intersectionality. *Canadian Public Policy, 44*(4), 306–316.

Harman, S. (2016). Ebola, gender and conspicuously invisible women in global health governance. *Third World Quarterly, 37*, 524–541.

Health Canada. (2020). *COVID-19 and sex, gender and intersectionality.* https://wiki.gccollab.ca/images/4/41/Guidance_Document_%28Full_EN%29.pdf. Accessed 3 Aug 2020.

Heymann, D. L. (2013). How SARS was contained. *The New York Times.* http://www.nytimes.com/2013/03/15/opinion/global/how-sars-was-contained.html. Accessed 11 Nov 2016.

Horby, P. W., Pfeiffer, D., & Oshitani, H. (2013). Prospects for emerging infections in east and Southeast Asia 10 years after severe acute respiratory syndrome. *Emerging Infectious Diseases, 19*(6), 853–860.

IOM GMDAC. (2020). Migration data relevant for the COVID-19 pandemic. *Migration Data Portal.* June 26, 2020. https://migrationdataportal.org/themes/migration-data-relevant-covid-19-pandemic. Accessed 15 Jul 2020.

Jamieson, D. J., Theiler, R. N., & Rasmussen, S. A. (2006). Emerging infections and pregnancy. *Emerging Infectious Diseases, 12*(11), 1638–1643.

Johns Hopkins Coronavirus Resource Centre. (2020). *COVID-19 dashboard by the centre for systems science and engineering.* https://coronavirus.jhu.edu/map.html. Accessed 14 Aug 2020.

Johnstone, R., & Momani, B. (2020). Health ministries need to look at race, ethnicity and socio economic data to assess the pandemic toll. Gender-based analysis plus is the tool for it. *Policy Options*. https://policyoptions.irpp.org/magazines/june-2020/a-gba-case-for-understanding-the-impact-of-covid-19/. Accessed 10 Jul 2020

Karlberg, J., Chong, D. S. Y., & Lai, W. Y. Y. (2004). Do men have a higher case fatality rate of severe acute respiratory syndrome than women do? *American Journal of Epidemiology, 159*(3), 229–231.

Kim, G. J. S., & Jackson, J. (2014). *Ebola outbreak and outcry: Saving Thomas Eric Duncan.* Huffington post. https://www.huffpost.com/entry/ebola-outbreak-and-outcry_b_5943216. Accessed 12 Jan 2015.

Lebeaux, R. (2016). *Developing nations and disadvantaged populations: How the 2009 H1N1 influenza pandemic exacerbated disparities and inequities. Independent study project collection* https://digitalcollections.sit.edu/isp_collection/2429. Accessed 4 Aug 2020

Lee, H., & Miller, V. J. (2020). The disproportionate impact of COVID-19 on minority groups: A social justice concern. *Journal of Gerontological Social Work, 6*, 1–5.

Maunder, R. (2004). The experience of the 2003 SARS outbreak as traumatic stress among frontline healthcare workers in Toronto: Lessons learned. *Philosophical Transactions of the Royal Society of London. Series B: Biological Sciences, 359*, 1117–1125.

McLafferty, S. (2010). Placing pandemics: Geographical dimensions of vulnerability and spread. *Eurasian Geography and Economics, 51*(2), 143–161.

Migrant Data Portal. (2020). *Migration data relevant for the COVID-19 pandemic.* https://migrationdataportal.org/themes/migration-data-relevant-covid-19-pandemic#foot. Accessed 10 Aug 2020.

Millett, G. A., Jones, A. T., Benkeser, D., Baral, S., Mercer, L., Beyrer, C., Honermann, B., Lankiewicz, E., Mena, L., Crowley, J. S., & Sherwood, J. (2020). Assessing differential impacts of COVID-19 on Black communities. *Annals of Epidemiology, 47*, 37–44.

Morens, D. M., Taubenberger, J. K., & Fauci, A. S. (2009). The persistent legacy of the 1918 influenza virus. *New England Journal of Medicine, 361*(3), 225–229.

Nkangu, M. N., Olatunde, O. A., & Yaya, S. (2017). The perspective of gender on the Ebola virus using a risk management and population health framework: A scoping review. *Infectious Diseases of Poverty, 6*(1), 135.

Nunes, J. (2016). Ebola and the production of neglect in global health. *Third World Quarterly, 37*, 542–556.

Patton, C. (2005). *Last served? Gendering the HIV pandemic.* London: Taylor & Francis.

Pirtle, W. N. L. (2020). Racial capitalism: A fundamental cause of novel coronavirus (COVID-19) pandemic inequities in the United States. *Health Education & Behavior, 47*, 504–508.

Preworski, A. (2020). COVID-19: A magnifier of social inequality. *The Global.* https://theglobal.blog/2020/06/09/covid-19-a-magnifier-of-social-inequality/. Accessed 5 Aug 2020.

Public Health Agency of Canada. (2003). *Learning from SARS: Renewal of Public Health in Canada.* Ottawa: PHAC.

Purdie, A., Hawkes, S., Buse, K., Onarheim, K., Aftab, W., Low, N., & Tanaka, S. (2020). Sex, gender and COVID-19: Disaggregated data and health disparities. *BMJ Global Health.* https://blogs.bmj.com/bmjgh/2020/03/24/sex-gender-and-covid-19-disaggregated-data-and-health-disparities/. Accessed 4 Jun 2020

Richardson, E. T., Collins, S. E., Kung, T., Jones, J. H., Tram, K. H., Boggiano, V. L., Bekker, L. G., & Zolopa, A. R. (2014). Gender inequality and HIV transmission: A global analysis. *Journal of the International AIDS Society, 17*(1), 19035.

San Martin, R., Painho, M., & Cruz-Jesus, F. (2019). Addressing geospatial preparedness inequity: A sustainable bottom-up approach for non-governmental development organizations. *Sustainability, 11*(23), 6634.

Schmidt, R. (2016). What does Zika have to do with equality? Everything. *Open Democracy.* https://www.opendemocracy.net/en/openglobalrights-openpage/what-does-zika-have-to-do-with-inequality-everything/. Accessed 1 Jun 2020 Office of the High Commissioner for Human Rights (2016) Upholding women's human rights essential to Zika response—Zeid. 5 February 2016. www.ohchr.org/EN/NewsEvents/Pages/DisplayNews. aspx?NewsID=17014&LangID=E; Accessed 10 Aug 2020

Schwalbe, N., Lehtimaki, S., & Gutierrez, J. P. (2020). *COVID-19: Rethinking risk, Lancet* https:// doi.org/10.1016/S2214-109X(20)30276-X. Accessed 5 Aug 2020

Smith, J. (2019). Overcoming the "tyranny of the urgent": Integrating gender into disease outbreak preparedness and response. *Gender and Development, 27*, 355–369.

Smith, J. (2020). Gender and the coronavirus outbreak. *Think Global Health*. https://www.think-globalhealth.org/article/gender-and-coronavirus-outbreak. Accessed 3 Aug 2020

Stern, A. M. (2016). Zika and reproductive justice. *Cadernos de Saude Publica*, 32(5) Epub June 3.

UN Women. (2014). *Ebola outbreak takes its toll on women*. 2 September 2014. https://www. unwomen.org/en/news/stories/2014/9/ebola-outbreak-takes-its-toll-on-women. Accessed 4 Aug 2020.

UN Women Inter-Agency Standing Committee, Reference Group for Gender in Humanitarian Action. (2015). *Humanitarian crisis in West Africa (Ebola) gender alert: February 2015* https://interagencystandingcommittee.org/system/files/iasc_gender_reference_group_-_gender_alert_west_africa_ebola_2_-_february_2015_0.pdf. Accessed 15 Jul 2020.

Vittor, A. Y. (2016). To tackle the Zika virus, alleviate urban poverty. *The New York Times* http:// www.nytimes.com/roomfordebate/2016/01/29/how-to-stop-the-spread-of-zika/to-tackle-the-zika-virus-alleviate-urban-poverty. Accessed 9 Feb 2016.

Watts, J. (2016). Brazil's sprawling favelas bear the brunt of the Zika epidemic. *The Guardian*. https://www.theguardian.com/world/2016/feb/07/brazil-rich-zika-virus-poor. Accessed 10 Feb 2016.

Wenham, C., Smith, J., & Morgan, R. (2020). COVID-19: The gendered impacts of the outbreak. *Lancet, 395*(10227), 846–848.

WHO. (2014). *Avian influenza – Fact sheet*. http://www.who.int/mediacentre/factsheets/avian_influenza/en/. Accessed 17 Nov 2014.

WHO. (2015a). *Origins of the 2014 Ebola epidemic* http://www.who.int/csr/disease/ebola/one-year-report/virus-origin/en/. Accessed 15 Jun 2020.

WHO. (2015b). *Factors that contributed to undetected spread of the Ebola virus and impeded rapid containment*. http://www.who.int/csr/disease/ebola/one-year-report/factors/en/. Accessed 4 Mar 2016.

WHO. (2016a). *Zika Virus – Fact sheet*. http://www.who.int/mediacentre/factsheets/zika/en/. Accessed 10 Nov 2016.

WHO. (2016b). *El Niño may increase breeding grounds for mosquitoes spreading Zika virus*, WHO says. http://who.int/hac/crises/el-nino/22february2016/en/. Accessed 12 Nov 2016.

WHO. (2016c) *Zika virus and the Olympic and Paralympic Games Rio 2016*. http://www.who.int/mediacentre/news/statements/2016/zika-olympics/en/. Accessed 16 Nov 2016

Wright, T. (2020). COVID-19 has greater impact on women advocates say. *Canada's National Observer.* https://www.nationalobserver.com/2020/04/10/news/covid-19-has-greater-impact-women-advocates-say. Accessed 30 Jul 2020.

Part III
The Responsibilities of Public Health

Chapter 11
Sex- and Gender-Based Analysis and the Social Determinants of Health: Public Health, Human Rights and Incarcerated Youth

Malin Lindroth and Catrine Andersson

Introduction

In this chapter, we focus on a sex- and gender-based analysis (SGBA) concerning young people incarcerated in state institutions in Sweden. We identify and discuss specific areas concerning sexual and reproductive health and rights (SRHR) wherein normative assumptions affect incarcerated young people's sexual health and their access to sexual health services.

As indicated by Mikkonen and Raphael (2010), the social determinants of health include a variety of factors that influence health outcomes both positively and negatively. This chapter discusses specific social determinants of health, including income and income distribution, education, unemployment and job security, employment and working conditions, early childhood development, food insecurity, housing, social exclusion, social safety network, health services, aboriginal status, gender, race, and disability. Further, the World Health Organization (2020) recognizes the social determinants of health as "the conditions in which people are born, grow, work, live, and age, and the wider set of forces and systems shaping the conditions of daily life. These forces and systems include economic policies and systems, development agendas, social norms, social policies, and political systems" (ibid). There is a vast body of evidence that shows a clear relationship between poverty, deprivation, and health outcomes (see, e.g. Marmot & Wilkinson, 2005). The social determinants of health are also closely connected to fundamental human rights, and it has been suggested that it is necessary for the fields of public health and human rights to "identify the fundamental causes of health and human rights inequities

M. Lindroth (✉) · C. Andersson
Centre for Sexology and Sexuality Studies, Department of Social Work, Faculty of Health and Society, Malmö University, Malmö, Sweden
e-mail: malin.lindroth@mau.se

© Springer Nature Switzerland AG 2021
J. Gahagan, M. K. Bryson (eds.), *Sex- and Gender-Based Analysis in Public Health*, https://doi.org/10.1007/978-3-030-71929-6_11

such as economic structures, class, and racism and to conceive ways of addressing them" (Haigh et al., 2019).

The social determinants of health also impact sexual health outcomes for young adults worldwide. According to the report of the Guttmacher-Lancet Commission on sexual and reproductive health and rights for all, young adults is a population in need of improved services, since "many social, gender, cultural, and legal barriers prevent adolescents from obtaining high-quality sexual and reproductive health information and services" (Starrs et al., 2018, p. 2668). In addition, the Convention on the Rights of the Child (2013) is clear. The General comment no. 15 on the right to the enjoyment of the highest attainable standard of health (art. 24) stresses the recognition of equal rights related to sexual and reproductive health; and equal access to information, education, justice and security; including the elimination of all forms of sexual and gender-based violence (ibid). These statements underline that sexual health is a public health responsibility.

Public health responses that prevent sexual health disparities and that promote sexual health should be designed by governmental or other regional public health agencies. These SRHR efforts must focus on the health of various populations while at the same time addressing barriers to health interventions, including those related to sexual health. One way to formalize this obligation can be to add them to official statements by government public health agencies. In the case of Sweden, the Public Health Agency (2020) official statements stress that sexuality and reproductive health are important determinants for health and fundamental for people's experience of health and well-being. The agency also emphasizes how it is that societal norms on sexuality and gender have an impact on conditions and possibilities for sexual and reproductive health, and advocates for a norm critical approach in the work towards sexual and reproductive health and rights on equal terms for the entire population. A norm critical approach implies an awareness of how societal norms on, for instance, age, gender, race, class, sexual orientation, and ability are connected to sexuality and how they can affect conditions and possibilities for experiencing sexual health (Public Health Agency of Sweden, 2016). Studies show that in practice, the situation for incarcerated youth is continuously precarious when it comes to the design of appropriate sexual and reproductive health care (Lindroth, 2020; Public Health Agency of Sweden, 2018; Schindele & Lindroth, 2020).

Young People in Secure State Care Institutions in Sweden

The Institutions and Access to Health Care

Unlike many other countries, Sweden does not have youth prisons. Rather, approximately 1,000 young persons (under 21 years of age) experiencing psychosocial issues, substance misuse, and criminal behaviour are placed in secure state institutions throughout the country annually (Swedish National Board of Institutional Care, 2020a). Before being placed in one of these 22 institutions, young people will have already received non-residential care in their home municipalities or care in a foster home or open residential home. Only when such interventions prove insufficient are they placed at these secure institutions. Further, care is provided mainly under the terms of the Care of Young Persons (Special Provisions) Act (Government of Sweden, 2020a) and is intended to be planned together with the young person, their family, and social services (Swedish National Board of Institutional Care, 2020a). Some institutions also care for those under 18 years (approximately 70 individuals per year) who have committed serious criminal offenses (e.g. assault, manslaughter, murder, drug crimes, sexual assaults, or rape) and are sentenced to secure youth care under the Secure Youth Care Act (Government of Sweden, 2020b). In comparison, the environment and the activities in these secure state institutions are similar to juvenile detention facilities, detention centres, or correctional facilities in the United States, or as described by Anderson et al. (2001): "Detainees are locked inside the facility for varying intervals depending on the outcome of their court appearances. They sleep, eat, attend school classes, participate in sports and recreation activities, and perform daily chores in their living units. Facility regulations assure that the detained teens receive close supervision during all of these activities" (ibid, p. 342).

To the best of our knowledge, no specific public health interventions, in general or in relation to sexual health, are offered by the National Board of Institutional Care aimed at young people in these institutions. This is a particular problem as incarcerated youth are regarded as a vulnerable population by the Public Health Agency of Sweden (2018) in terms of sexual health. Regional and local public health care does not consider youth at secure institutions within their geographical area to be their responsibility. This "blind spot" in terms of responsibility for health care, in particular sexual and reproductive health care, for this group of young people is worrisome and adds to health inequality. With institutions often localized in secluded areas outside cities, the sexual health promotion needs of young people are overlooked by national, regional, and local healthcare authorities. This points to the importance of looking at the organization of care and responsibilities for vulnerable groups. First, a description of young people at these secure care institutions follows.

Young People at Secure Care Institutions, Their Social Determinants of Health and Actual Health

Young people between the ages of 16 and 29 in secure state care face greater socio-economic disadvantage as compared with their non-state care peers (Public Health Agency of Sweden, 2017, 2018; Ybrandt & Nordqvist, 2015). There is also an overrepresentation of young people with intellectual or neuropsychiatric disabilities (defined according to the DSM-IV diagnostic criteria for AD/HD, autism spectrum disorder, and mental retardation) at secure state institutions (Anckarsäter et al., 2008; Ståhlberg et al., 2010). This is worth noting since disability is an important social determinant of health (Mikkonen & Raphael, 2010). When compared to their same-aged non-incarcerated peers, young people in secure state care have parents with lower educational levels who may also have employment challenges and have higher rates of mental health problems, criminality, and substance use issues (Ybrandt & Nordqvist, 2015). Consequently, these young persons experience poor social and health outcomes (Kling et al., 2016; Schindele & Lindroth, 2020; Tordön et al., 2018; Vinnerljung & Sallnäs, 2008). The same applies to educational levels, perceived economic status, and mental health: young people in secure state care differ from their non-incarcerated peers (Public Health Agency of Sweden, 2017, 2018; Schindele & Lindroth, 2020). When young people at four secure Swedish state care homes underwent systematic medical exams several unknown or untreated health problems were discovered. Ninety-three per cent of the girls and 67 per cent of the boys needed referrals to somatic care, dental care, youth clinic (i.e. a public health sexual and reproductive health clinic), or vaccination within school health care (Kling et al., 2016).

In addition to these differences in access to health care and health outcomes, young people in secure state care also have worse sexual health outcomes (Lindroth et al., 2013; Public Health Agency of Sweden, 2017, 2018; Schindele & Lindroth, 2020). When sexual health risks and variables predicting adverse sexual health outcomes were compared between young people in secure state care in Sweden and their non-incarcerated same-aged peers, major differences were found (ibid). Specifically, young people in secure state care had higher rates of chlamydia, experienced sexual assault, and had unprotected (no birth control or condom) vaginal or anal intercourse the last time they had sex (ibid).

It is important to note that sexual behaviour, poor sexual health, or the risk for poor sexual health outcomes is not a prerequisite for placement in secure state care. However, young people who have committed sexual crimes and been sentenced to care under the Secure Youth Care Act are placed in secure state care, although the number of individuals placed in secure state care is low. In 2016, nine young persons (under the age of 20) were sentenced to secure state care due to sexual offenses (Swedish National Board of Institutional Care, 2017). All young people, including those who have committed sexual crimes, have the right to sexual health promotion information and knowledge, for instance, thorough comprehensive sex education and the right to contraception counselling and testing during their placement according to the Education Act (Government of Sweden, 2020c). The general lack of training and specific lack of competence within the field of sexual and reproductive health and rights among staff is a major drawback hypothesized to result in institutional gaps and silences surrounding sexuality and sexual health needs (Lindroth, 2020; Överlien, 2004). Accordingly, sexual health promotion needs are evident, and a sex- and gender-based analysis that takes the specific needs of this population into account is vital.

A Sex- and Gender-Based Analysis of Incarcerated Young People and Their Right to Sexual Health

In the following section, we apply a sex- and gender-based analysis to public health obligations to support rights to sexual health for young people in incarceration. We focus on five specific areas where normative assumptions affect incarcerated young people's access to sexual health services: gender-stereotypical norms within secure care institutions; heteronormative organization of care; cis-normativity and general lack of transgender and non-binary competent care and caregivers; ideas of normalcy in relation to young people and sexuality and SRHR competence in secure care.

Gender-stereotypical norms among staff that affect young people within secure care institutions have been described in a number of ethnographic studies (Henriksen, 2018; Laanemets and Kristiansen, 2008). Young men's expressions of sexuality and intimacy have historically been unproblematized and explained as biologically expected behaviours while the opposite has been the case for young women. Their expressions of sexuality and intimacy were understood as femininity connected to their bodies, and female sexuality and bodies seen as commodities in need of protection (Laanemets and Kristiansen, 2008). Differences in practices used for disciplining girls and boys in secure care have been described as follows: "boys are disciplined to promote working-class masculinity; girls are disciplined to promote normative femininity and contained heterosexuality" (Henriksen, 2018, p. 440). This implies that young women, as opposed to young men, are made responsible for their sexuality while incarcerated, regardless of whether or not previous sexual experiences are a reason for their placement. These normative assumptions among staff have also been described by Överlien (2004) in an ethnographic study at a secure institution specialized in caring for young women with experiences of sexual violence. Researchers in this area have documented how staff typically regard young women as sexually destructive and in need of protection from sexuality, both their own and male staff members' sexuality. Young women are seen to be in need of a "rest from sexuality," since this rest could provide them with the opportunity to restore their sexuality from dysfunctional and inappropriate to healthy and normal (Överlien, 2004, p. 72). A more recent ethnographic study found that young women in secure state care have been seen through a lens of victimization, but that this lens is inconsistent with the young women's self-described identities, as they do not recognize or typically see themselves as victims (Vogel, 2017). Young men also stand to lose from normative assumptions since a working-class masculinity ideal is not a fit for all young men. While young women as well as young men and gender non-binary youth need to be protected from sexual violence, there are risks involved in basing secure care too heavily in an approach of protection and risks. Sheltering young people and letting them "rest" from sexuality can be strategies where expressions of sexuality are silenced. Instead, a public health approach to sexual health and *rights* could be a way forward.

We do not suggest that the cisnormative, gender-stereotypical, heteronormative assumptions or processes described earlier are specific to secure state care institutions. Rather, they are a part of society in general and are reflected in all facets of social institutions, including within secure state care institutions. In addition, they are also a part of the very organization of secure state care, with gender-segregated institutions or wards aiming to minimize sexual relations between young people. Commuting between worlds—the institution, where sexuality should be abstained from, and the outside world, where sexuality may be a part of every day—can be demanding for both the young person and for the staff (Lindroth, 2020). Secondly, two out of ten young persons (16–29 years) placed in secure state care define themselves outside of heterosexual norms. In particular, 28 per cent of the young women and 2 per cent of the young men identify as bisexual (Public Health Agency of Sweden, 2018), compared to 7 per cent of young women and 3 per cent of young men 16–29 years of age in the general population (Public Health Agency of Sweden, 2017).

The high number of young women in secure state care who identify as bisexual is important to note in relation to previous international studies indicating that women who have sex with both women and men are particularly vulnerable regarding sexual health and general health overall (e.g. Mercer et al., 2007). A recent Swedish survey of SRHR in the population also found young bisexual women to be a particularly vulnerable group (Public Health Agency of Sweden, 2017). Overrepresentation of queer youth has similarly been observed in U.S. juvenile justice facilities, where the number of incarcerated young girls who identify as bisexual or lesbian (39 per cent) significantly exceeds the prevalence in the general population (12 per cent). This identification as queer renders young people simultaneously invisible and hypervisible in the juvenile justice system (Mountz, 2020; Robinson, 2020).

The issue of gender-separated wards as discussed earlier is further problematized by bringing gender identities into the analysis. In a national survey of sexuality and health amongst young people in Sweden, one per cent identified themselves as being or having been transgender, and one per cent elected not to categorize their gender (Public Health Agency of Sweden, 2017). When the same survey was aimed at young people in secure state care, no one identified as transgender or non-binary (Public Health Agency of Sweden, 2018). However, the issue is not merely one of numbers, but of responsibilities regarding preventive measures. Since transgender and gender non-binary identities are connected to the risk of discrimination, they are important social determinants of health (Public Health Agency of Sweden, 2015, 2016). This places an obligation on the state authority running secure state institutions to design care, e.g. access to private spaces that are not designated for either young women or young men only or sex education that is not cis-normative. In addition, staff working at the institutions need to be knowledgeable regarding transgender and non-binary gender identities. Studies show that low awareness and education regarding transgender and non-binary genders results in a higher risk of professionals seeking information from the transgender or non-gender individuals seeking care, resulting in them experiencing being "a live teaching material," "a dictionary," or always "the one who teaches in your everyday life" (Lindroth, 2016, p. 3516). Interventions considering these aspects of gender variability provide an example of how to tailor secure state care by means of the application of an SGBA lens.

Sexual health promotion interventions aimed at young people in secure state care exist. However, they are rare, and not free from gender-stereotypical assumptions, and lack a positive approach to youth sexuality, and they tend not to be designed with a human rights-based perspective (Hammarström et al., 2018). Public health interventions from a critical perspective would benefit from taking sexuality-related concerns such as pleasure, rights, autonomy, freedom, and desire into consideration (Epstein & Mamo, 2017). Issues of sexual and reproductive *rights* are central for avoiding current tendencies to regulate youth sexuality in relation to social norms that prioritize the avoidance of risky behaviours and encouragement of "normal" sexuality, especially in girls. As discussed throughout this chapter, staff competencies in SGBA and SRHR are crucial components for addressing issues of sexual health with a public health and sexual rights perspective. Young people in state care risk being housed with staff who lack training and education regarding gender, sexuality, and other social determinants of health. A person who lacks education about SRHR and human rights in the context of youth work is left to base their judgements on their personal values, experiences, and knowledge. It is hypothesized that invisibility and silence surrounding sexuality and sexual health issues in secure institutions are connected to a lack of staff competence and that the silence is further upheld by both staff and young persons but for different reasons. Young people keep quiet about health needs for fear of being judged by staff (see Lindroth, 2020). However, efforts are being made, and good examples exist. In 2018, the National Board of Institutional Care in cooperation with an NGO, the Swedish Association for Sexuality Education, launched a series of four web-educations for staff working at the secure care institutions (Swedish National Board of Institutional Care, 2020b). The education covered (1) the introduction to SRHR for all staff (e.g. social workers, nurses, psychologists, physicians, and administrative staff), (2) SRHR for nurses, (3) SRHR for the school health team, and (4) SRHR for staff working specifically with substance abuse treatment. It remains to be seen how well implemented and sustainable this public health effort is in improving the sexual health outcomes of young people in care.

Concluding Remarks

Governments and related public health agencies must assure, on both policy and practice levels, that inequalities in access to sexual health care and related sexual health outcomes for incarcerated young people are addressed. In Sweden, policies exist, including the use of a sex- and gender-based analysis, but clear action on the practice level is lacking. The national Public Health Agency has addressed young people in secure state care as a group in need of interventions, but in light of the analysis in this chapter, we see several challenges that need to be addressed: (1) the lack of SRHR competence in staff, (2) the organization of sexual and reproductive health care being unclear and risking the accessibility for incarcerated youth, and (3) the organization of secure state care building on gender-stereotypical, heteronormative, and cis-normative ideas of youth sexualities and identities, which risks emphasizing existing vulnerabilities. This is evident in both the case of gender-separated wards and the implicit ideas of youth sexualities and identities that organize the care. Public health at all levels has a key role to play in working concretely to address the sex- and gender-based challenges to sexual health outcomes of youth in secure care as outlined in this chapter.

References

Anckarsäter, H., Nilsson, T., Saury, J.-M., Råstam, M., & Gillberg, C. (2008). Autism spectrum disorders in institutionalized subjects. *Nordic Journal of Psychiatry, 62*(2), 160–167.

Anderson, N. L., Nyamathi, A., McAvoy, J. A., Conde, F., & Casey, C. (2001). Perceptions about risk for HIV/AIDS among adolescents in juvenile detention. *Western Journal of Nursing Research, 23*(4), 336–359.

Convention on the Rights of the Child. (2013). *General comment No. 15 (2013) on the right of the child to the enjoyment of the highest attainable standard of health (art. 24).* United Nations: Committee on the rights of the child.

Epstein, S., & Mamo, L. (2017). The proliferation of sexual health: Diverse social problems and the legitimation of sexuality. *Social Science & Medicine, 188*, 176–190.

Government of Sweden. (2020a). *Care of young persons (special provisions) act (1990:52).* Retrieved 2020-05-20 from: https://www.riksdagen.se/sv/dokument-lagar/dokument/ svensk-forfattningssamling/lag-199052-med-sarskilda-bestammelser-om-vard_sfs-1990-52

Government of Sweden. (2020b). *Care of young persons (special provisions) act (1998:603).* Retrieved 2020-05-20 from: https://www.riksdagen.se/sv/dokument-lagar/dokument/ svensk-forfattningssamling/lag-1998603-om-verkstallighet-av-sluten_sfs-1998-603

Government of Sweden. (2020c). *Education act (2010:800).* Retrieved 2020-05-20 from: https://www.riksdagen.se/sv/dokument-lagar/dokument/svensk-forfattningssamling/ skollag-2010800_sfs-2010-800

Haigh, F., Kemp, L., Bazeley, P., & Haigh, N. (2019). Developing a critical realist informed framework to explain how the human rights and social determinants of health relationship works. *BMC Public Health, 19*, 1571. https://doi.org/10.1186/s12889-019-7760-7

Hammarström, S., Stenquist, K., & Lindroth, M. (2018). Sexual health interventions for young people in state care: A systematic review. *Scandinavian Journal of Public Health, 46*(8), 817–834.

Henriksen, A.-K. (2018). Vulnerable girls and dangerous boys: Gendered practices of discipline in secure care. *Young, 26*(5), 427–443.

Kling, S., Vinnerljung, B., & Hjern, A. (2016). *Hälsokontroll för SiS-ungdomar. En studie av hälsoproblem och vårdbehov hos ungdomar på fyra särskilda ungdomshem.* Stockholm: Statens institutionsstyrelse.

Laanemets L & Kristiansen, A. (2008). Kön och behandling inom tvångsvård – En studie av hur vården organiseras med avseende på genus. [Gender and care in compulsory care–A study of how care is organized regarding gender] Stockholm: The Swedish National Board of Institutional Care.

Lindroth M, Tikkanen R & Löfgren-Mårtenson L. 2013. Unequal sexual health-Differences between detained youth and their same-aged peers. Scandinavian Journal of Public Health, 41(7), 720–726.

Lindroth, M. (2016). "Competent persons who can treat you with competence, as simple as that" – an interview study with transgender people on their experiences of meeting health care professionals. Journal of Clinical Nursing, 23–24, 3511–3521.

Lindroth, M. (2020). On the outskirts of the charmed circle – Challenges and limitations of sexual health promotion to young people in secure state care. Sexuality Research and Social Policy, 1–10. https://doi.org/10.1007/s13178-020-00433-1

Marmot, M., & Wilkinson, R. G. (2005). Social determinants of health. Oxford Scholarship Online. https://doi.org/10.1093/acprof:oso/9780198565895.001.0001.

Mercer, C. H., Bailey, J. V., Johnson, A. M., Erens, B., Wellings, K., Fenton, K. A., & Copas, A. J. (2007). Women who report having sex with women: British national probability data on prevalence, sexual behaviors, and health outcomes. American Journal of Public Health, 97(6), 1126–1133. https://doi.org/10.2105/AJPH.2006.086439

Mikkonen, J., & Raphael, D. (2010). Social determinants of health: The Canadian facts. Toronto: York University School of Health Policy and Management.

Mountz, S. (2020). Remapping pipelines and pathways: Listening to queer and transgender youth of color's trajectories through girls' juvenile justice facilities. Affilia, 35(2), 177–199. https://doi.org/10.1177/0886109919880517

Överlien, C. (2004). Girls on the verge of exploding? Voices on sexual abuse, agency and sexuality at a youth detention home. Doctoral dissertation. Linköping: Linköping University.

Public Health Agency of Sweden (2015). Health and health determinants among transgender persons – A report on the health status of transgender persons in Sweden. In Swedish, summary in English available at: https://www.folkhalsomyndigheten.se/publicerat-material/publikationsarkiv/h/halsan-och-halsans-bestamningsfaktorer-for-transpersoner-en-rapport-om-halsolaget-bland-transpersoner-i-sverige/

Public Health Agency of Sweden. (2016). The right to health – How norms and structures affect transgender people's experiences of sexual health. In Swedish, summary in English. Available at: https://www.folkhalsomyndigheten.se/contentassets/3b29bf7ea68948c6af3e6b92b2ac524a/ratten-halsa-16045-webb.pdf

Public Health Agency of Sweden. (2017). Sexuality and health among young people in Sweden. Stockholm: Folkhälsomyndigheten. In Swedish, summary in English. Available at: https://www.folkhalsomyndigheten.se/contentassets/11272529714342b390d40fe3200f48cf/sexualitet-halsa-bland-unga-sverige-01186-2017-1-webb.pdf

Public Health Agency of Sweden. (2018). Sexualitet och hälsa bland unga och unga vuxnainom statlig institutionsvård [Sexuality and health among young people and young adults in secure state care]. Stockholm: Folkhälsomyndigheten.

Public Health Agency of Sweden. (2020). Retrieved 2020-05-05 from: https://www.folkhalsomyndigheten.se/the-public-health-agency-of-sweden/living-conditions-and-lifestyle/sexual-health/

Robinson, B. A. (2020). The lavender scare in homonormative times: Policing, hyper-incarceration, and LGBTQ youth homelessness. Gender & Society, 34(2), 210–232. https://doi.org/10.1177/0891243220906172

Schindele, A. C. C., & Lindroth, M. (2020). Sexual and reproductive health and rights (SRHR) among young people in secure state care and their non-incarcerated peers – A qualitative, descriptive and comparative study. European Journal of Social Work, 1–4. https://doi.org/10.1080/13691457.2020.1815658

Ståhlberg, O., Anckarsäter, H., & Nilsson, T. (2010). Mental health problems in youths committed to juvenile institutions: Prevalences and treatment needs. European Child & Adolescent Psychiatry, 19(12), 893–903.

Starrs, A. M., Ezeh, A. C., Barker, G., Basu, A., Bertrand, J. T., Blum, R., Coll-Seck, A. M., et al. (2018). Accelerate progress—Sexual and reproductive health and rights for all: Report of the Guttmacher–lancet commission. The Lancet, 391(10140), 2642–2692.

Swedish National Board of Institutional Care. (2017). *SiS i korthet 2016. En samling statistiska uppgifter om SiS. [SiS briefly 2016. A collection of statistical information on SiS]*. Stockholm: Statens institutionsstyrelse.

Swedish National Board of Institutional Care. (2020a). Retrieved 2020-05-05 from: https://www.stat-inst.se/var-verksamhet/halso-och-sjukvard/

Swedish National Board of Institutional Care. (2020b). *SiS Årsredovisning 2018. [SiS Annual Report 2018]* Retrieved 2020-07-07 from: https://www.stat-inst.se/globalassets/arsredovisningar/arsredovisning-2018.pdf

Tordön, R., Svedin, C. G., Fredlund, C., Jonsson, L., Priebe, G., & Sydsjö, G. (2018). Background, experiences of abuse and mental health among adolescents in out-of-home care: A cross-sectional study of a Swedish high school national sample. *Nordic Journal of Psychiatry, 73*(1), 16–23.

Vinnerljung, B., & Sallnäs, M. (2008). Into adulthood: A follow-up study of 718 young people who were placed in out-of-home care during their teens. *Child and Family Social Work, 13*, 144–155.

Vogel, M. A. (2017). Endeavour for autonomy – How girls understand their lived experiences of being referred to secure care. *YOUNG. Nordic Journal of Youth Research, 26*(1), 70–85.

World Health Organization. (2020). Retrieved 2020-05-05 from: https://www.who.int/social_determinants/en/

Ybrandt, H., & Nordqvist, S. (2015). *SiS-placerade ungdomars problematik i relation till andra ungdomar. [SiS-placed youth and their problems in relation to other youth]*. Stockholm: Statens Institutionsstyrelses.

Chapter 12
Gender-Transformative Public Health Approaches

Olena Hankivsky and Gemma Hunting

Introduction

It is well-established that gender inequalities drive inequities in health and well-being (Annandale & Hunt, 2000; EuroHealthNet, 2017; Hawkes et al., 2020; Hawkes & Buse, 2013; Heise et al., 2019; Sen & Östlin, 2007). Gender, a social construct, is embedded within and across organizations, systemic structures, and institutional norms. A mounting body of evidence also highlights that gender norms are key drivers of gender inequality and health inequity shaping differential exposure to health risks, health-related behaviours and access to care but are not always recognized or addressed (Heise et al., 2019; Darmstadt et al., 2019; Hawkes et al., 2020). The growing acknowledgement of this reality is transforming the entire landscape of public health, including the development and strengthening of mainstream frameworks and tools such as gender-transformative approaches (GTA).[1] This is evidenced by GTA examples that explicitly mention or try to integrate intersectionality and the

---

[1] The term "gender-transformative approach" was first coined by Gupta (2000) in relation to addressing HIV/AIDS and has gained particular traction in global health and development (Ruane-McAteer et al., 2019). It is important to note that gender-transformative approaches (GTA) to improve health come from a wide variety of disciplines, including public health, global health, psychology, social work, and epidemiology. Given this, a number of different disciplinary frameworks shape specific gender-transformative approaches and interventions (Dworkin & Barker, 2019). Given the scope of this chapter, we offer a review of general trends related to public health-focused GTA models and frameworks in relation to intersectionality, rather than a comprehensive analysis of gender-transformative approaches, models, or interventions.

O. Hankivsky (✉)
Centre for Health Equity, Melbourne School of Population and Global Health, University of Melbourne, Carlton, VIC, Australia
e-mail: o.hankivsky@unimelb.edu.au

G. Hunting
International Health Equity Consultant, Coburg, Bavaria, Germany

© Springer Nature Switzerland AG 2021   149
J. Gahagan, M. K. Bryson (eds.), *Sex- and Gender-Based Analysis in Public Health*, https://doi.org/10.1007/978-3-030-71929-6_12

development, in the Canadian context, of sex- and gender-based analysis plus (SGBA+), which is an explicit attempt to integrate intersectionality.

The inclusion of intersectionality within GTA represents important developments in terms of advancing gender equality and health equity. However, current GTAs do not yet reflect the true potential of intersectionality to transform public health. Arguably, the *interplay* of the full range of complex factors and influencing forces and structures of power that underpin health inequities is not adequately accounted for. Specifically, what is needed is a more robust analysis and concrete action to understand experiences of health inequities, who is at disproportionate risk, the differences between groups of people at disproportionate risk, and how appropriate population health responses can be crafted and targeted to social groups most at risk. Only then can the ultimate goal of GTA – to transform power inequities – be fully realized.

Background: Gender-Transformative Approaches

Many different definitions of gender-transformative approaches, applied to both health and social contexts, have been offered to date. For example, gender-transformative health approaches are commonly defined as able "to reshape gender relations to be more gender equitable, largely through approaches that free both women and men from the impact of destructive gender and sexual norms" (Gupta, 2000, p. 6; Fleming et al., 2014; Greaves et al., 2014; WHO, 2011). Rolleri (2014, p. 3) describes that gender transformative interventions aim to (1) raise awareness about unhealthy gender norms, (2) question the costs of adhering to these norms, and (3) replace unhealthy, inequitable gender norms with redefined healthy ones. It has been asserted that a GTA actively examines, questions, and changes rigid gender norms and imbalances of power (Fleming et al., 2014; Rutgers, 2020; Rottach et al., 2009).

And while it is also the case that great variation exists in how GTA interventions have been implemented, there are some key interrelated aspirations of GTA, namely, that they are designed to:

- Challenge gender norms and inequality at multiple levels – from individual to societal – to improve social conditions for women and girls.
- Encourage awareness of inequitable gender roles and norms and the advantages of addressing them for society.
- Empower and strengthen the agency of women and girls.
- Engage boys and men in gender equality and its benefits for society.
- Consider diversity (e.g. gender, sexual identity) when addressing the needs of women, men, boys, and girls.

(Adapted from: Rutgers, 2018; Plan International, 2019)

The ultimate goal of transformative and sustainable change has been described as focusing on three dimensions of empowerment: (1) agency, individual and collective capacities (knowledge and skills), attitudes, critical reflection, assets, actions, and access to services; (2) relations, the expectations and cooperative or negotiation dynamics embedded within relationships between people in the home, market, community, and groups and organizations; and (3) structures, the informal and formal institutional rules that govern collective, individual, and institutional practices, such as environment, social norms, recognition, and status (Martinez & Wu, 2009; Morgan, 2014).

In the context of health, it has been asserted that GTA seek to move beyond a focus on "risk groups" and individual-level behaviours to focus on restructuring power relationships that create and maintain gender inequalities (Dworkin & Barker, 2019; Fleming et al., 2014; Hillenbrand et al., 2015; Trickett et al., 2011). More recent conceptualizations and frameworks of GTA go so far as to claim that they recognize the importance of intersectionality and address intersecting factors, which may amplify gender inequalities, such as class, caste differences, race, ethnic descent, different (dis)abilities, age, and schooling (e.g. Rutgers, 2018; SGBA+ in Canada).

Intersectionality

The potential of intersectionality has increasingly been recognized as both complementary and necessary for gender-transformative research (Fehrenbacher & Patel, 2020; Peretz et al., 2020; Rutgers, 2020; WHO, 2020). Specifically, it facilitates an examination of the multiple and interacting power dynamics that maintain gender and intersecting inequalities, reflecting increasing international consensus that looking at gender or gender inequality alone is inefficient to address social and health inequities (e.g. UN Women, 2020).

The term "intersectionality" was coined in 1989 by American critical legal race scholar Kimberlé Williams Crenshaw (1989), but the central ideas of intersectionality have long historic roots within and beyond the United States. Black activists and feminists, as well as Latina, post-colonial, queer, and Indigenous scholars have all produced work that reveals the complex factors and processes that shape human lives (Bunjun, 2010; Chan et al., 2019; Collins, 1990; Collins & Bilge, 2016; Grzanka & Grzanka, 2018; Hancock, 2016; Roth, 2018; Valdes, 1997; Van Herk et al., 2011).

Put succinctly, intersectionality posits that inequities are never the result of single, distinct factors. Rather, there are many factors that interact to influence any one person, their life, experiences, and needs.

> Intersectionality promotes an understanding of human beings as shaped by the interaction of different social locations (e.g. "race"/ethnicity, Indigeneity, gender, class, sexuality, geography, age, disability/ability, migration status, religion). These interactions occur within a context of connected systems and structures of power (e.g. laws, policies, state governments and other political and economic unions, religious institutions, media). Through such processes, interdependent forms of privilege and oppression shaped by colonialism, imperialism, racism, homophobia, ableism, and patriarchy are created. (Hankivsky, 2014, p. 2)

Key tenets of an intersectionality approach include the following:

- Human lives cannot be explained by taking into account single categories, such as gender, race, and socioeconomic status. People's lives are multidimensional and complex. Lived realities are shaped by different factors and social dynamics operating together. Understanding their interaction goes beyond simply adding together several factors. It is focused on their interactions.
- When analysing health and social issues, the importance of any category or structure cannot be predetermined; the categories and their importance must be discovered in the process of investigating a problem or phenomenon.
- Relationships and power dynamics between social locations (gender, race, and socioeconomic status) and processes (e.g. racism, classism, heterosexism, ableism, ageism, sexism) are linked. They can also change over time and be different depending on geographic location. Multilevel analyses that link individual experiences to broader structures and systems are crucial for revealing how power relations are shaped and experienced.
- People can experience discrimination and privilege simultaneously. This depends on what situation or specific context they are in. While people can experience different forms of vulnerability, they also have agency and different sources of resilience to respond to their situations.
- Scholars, researchers, policy-makers, and activists must consider their own social position, role, and power when taking an intersectional approach. This "reflexivity" should be in place before setting priorities and directions in research, policy work, and activism.
- Intersectionality is explicitly oriented towards transformation, building coalitions among different groups, and working towards social justice (adapted from Hankivsky, 2014, p. 3).

Intersectionality and Public Health

The importance of intersectionality in the context of public health is widely recognized. In her 2012 seminal article, Bowleg argued:

> Public health's commitment to social justice makes it a natural fit with intersectionality's focus on multiple historically oppressed populations. Yet despite a plethora of research focused on these populations, public health studies that reflect intersectionality in their theoretical frameworks, designs, analyses, or interpretations are rare. (p. 1267)

Intersectionality-informed approaches align with and complement the core principles of public health, such as a commitment to social justice, an emphasis on structural interventions, and a focus on community-based participatory action research (Thomas et al., 2002). In the last decade, public health researchers have started to not only highlight but also demonstrate how intersectionality helps to reveal the interplay of root causes of health inequities and, in particular, the interaction of structures and systems of power such as patriarchy, racism, homophobia, ableism, ageism, and how they interact with multiple and simultaneous identities for diverse individuals within the population (Gkiouleka et al., 2018; Hankivsky & Christoffersen, 2008; Kapilashrami et al., 2015; Kapilashrami & Hankivsky, 2018; Krieger, 2014).

Intersectionality and Gender-Transformative Approaches to Public Health

Intersectionality has been argued to be well-suited for gender-transformative approaches to public health because (1) it challenges models that operationalize social determinants of health as distinct, unchanging categories and (2) it provides a framework for understanding the interlocking effects of different identities and social structures on health (Fehrenbacher & Patel, 2020; Greaves et al., 2014). A recent scoping review of gender-transformative health promotion frameworks in 2019 describes intersectionality as a common principle of such frameworks (Horgan et al., 2020), and many key public and global health practitioners are drawing from intersectionality in their GTA work (Dworkin & Barker, 2019).

For example, Pederson et al. (2014) developed a "framework for gender transformative health promotion" to model how gender transformation should be an explicit aim of health promotion practice, policy-making, and research (CEWH, 2020). The framework incorporates "gendered health determinants" – biological, environmental, social, political, cultural, and economic factors – which interact to create gendered social structures and systems. The framework entails looking at how multiple factors intersect with sex and gender (considered "fundamental determinants of health") to shape differential health and social outcomes for women.

Another promising development is the innovative model developed by the government of Canada – sex- and gender-based analysis plus (SGBA+), modelled on GBA+, which is called "gender transformative" and is intended to break down systemic barriers to reach true gender equality. GBA+ has been described as the federal government's response to the growing diversity of Canada's population and the need for an evolution in GBA that could address gender along with other identity factors for diverse groups of women and men and girls and boys (SCSW, 2016).

Fig. 12.1 Government of
Canada's approach: GBA+
(Status of Women Canada,
2018)

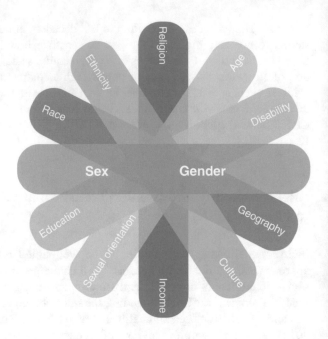

GBA+ (Fig. 12.1) is designed to consider many factors – in addition to gender – like race, ethnicity, religion, age, and mental or physical disability. SGBA+, being used by the Institute for Gender and Health within the Canadian Institutes of Health Research, recognizes intersecting factors in addition to sex and gender. SGBA+ is also considered an important tool to aid the creation and evaluation of public health prevention and health promotion efforts to determine the extent to which they implement a gender-transformative approach or promote inclusivity in relation to populations that experience sex, gender, and intersectional inequities (Stinson et al., 2020).

While approaches to GTA that attempt to connect gender equality with an intersectional view of inequalities between women and men and girls and boys are important developments, there are ways in which they fall short of the requirements of intersectionality. Specifically, they give primal focus to sex and gender (and most often, women). The fact remains that most approaches, including those discussed earlier, defend gender (and sex) as *the* logical entry points for acknowledging and openly discussing multiple forms of inequity. This has far-reaching implications.

First, GTA health models often fall into the trap of advancing binary conceptions of gender (Dworkin & Barker, 2019; Dworkin et al., 2015) and the conflation of sex with gender. For instance, the discourse and focus is predominantly on outdated constructs of women (mostly) and/or men (less commonly) who are assumed to fulfil binary cisgender notions of femaleness and maleness. This eclipses the experiences of gender- and sex-diverse populations and ignores how gender, gender identities, masculinities, and femininities, as social constructions, can change across time and context.

In addition, despite a focus on gender transformation to benefit the health of all, few gender-transformative frameworks and initiatives explicitly focus on how men might benefit from such approaches (e.g. Horgan et al., 2020). In fact, most focus on issues of gender-based violence (GBV) and/or maternal and child health. This can undermine the efficacy and take-up of GTAs because of the perception that these approaches are only relevant to women and in specific niche areas of concern (Horgan et al., 2020).

Further, attention to intersectionality is an add-on or integration, with a strong assumption that with changes in norms and behaviours will come changes in the interconnected social relations that foster and reinforce gender-based health inequities. Experience with gender analysis and gender mainstreaming efforts, however, has shown that this does not automatically follow (George et al., 2020; Sen & Östlin, 2007).

Not surprisingly, Fehrenbacher and Patel (2020) have argued that GTA health frameworks that acknowledge the importance of intersectionality prioritize gender, gender norms, and institutions at the expense of other factors and process and structures of power. Dworkin et al. (2015) have similarly concluded that GTAs do not go far enough to capture the root causes of a problem, produce difficulties in maintaining long-term positive intervention effects, or lead to unintended consequences.

Such critiques have led Fehrenbacher and Patel (2020) to argue that while "gender transformation provides a useful entry point for intersectional health research and should always be assessed… gender *need not be* the focal stratifier of every study depending on the research question or goal of an intervention" (emphasis added, p. 147). This is true for GTA, specifically, but also in public health research more generally. Intersectionality is often conflated with gender analysis; researchers tend to focus on select and distinct variables (rather than interactive processes) and also fail to understand the complexities of health inequities as well as the importance of resilience and resistance (Rosenthal, 2016).

In contrast, intersectionality recognizes that experiences of inequity are shaped by gendered forces and factors that intersect and are co-constituted by other diverse factors. These dynamics change across time and place; gender may not be most salient in a given context for an individual or group. Thus, starting with gender or women a priori in GTA may overlook more salient factors influencing inequity in a given situation or context. When inequities are understood as not being restricted to gender but as inseparable from other factors such as class, race/ethnicity, sexuality, immigration status, geography, and ability – without any presumption of ranking – this has profound implications for understandings of human lives, experience, and concomitant inequities.

Realizing the Potential of Intersectionality in GTA: Next Steps

If gender-transformative approaches can truly explore and gain from the health equity-promoting potential of intersectionality, some key concrete actions and changes are required.

First, there will need to be more accurate operationalization of intersectionality in the context of GTAs and public health more generally (Fehrenbacher & Patel, 2020; Heard et al., 2020). This ultimately requires exploring and understanding the full implication of intersectionality for existing GTAs and the processes involved in their uptake and operationalization. Guidance for doing this work includes the *Intersectionality-Based Policy Analysis (IBPA) Framework* (Hankivsky et al., 2012), which provides principles and guiding questions grounded in intersectionality to help highlight and address relevant equity dynamics in various health-relevant disciplines and sectors.[2]

Next, further empirical research on the interrelationships between different axes of social power and oppression, including but not limited to gender and its impact on health, is needed to create gender-transformative interventions and policies. In particular, there is a need to develop innovative methods of data collection that capture complex relationships between individual and societal levels (Bowleg, 2012; Hankivsky, 2014).

Lastly, and more generally, there is a need to develop and strengthen approaches to transformative change in health and social inequities, requiring more engagement with intersectionality-informed methodologies in qualitative, quantitative, and mixed methods and specifically policy-focused research to challenge well-entrenched power structures and processes that shape public health – something that GTAs aspire to change. Combined, such efforts can inform public health interventions and policies that address the root causes of health inequities and reveal and challenge power structures through attention to the contextual, complex, and relational aspects of health and well-being (Hankivsky et al., 2017).

---

[2] The IBPA Framework has been recognized as a promising health equity tool (e.g. Buettgen et al., 2018; Heard et al., 2020; Mendell et al., 2012; Palència et al., 2014; NCCHPP, 2015) and has been taken up across a wide array of health-relevant fields including violence, mental health and substance use, HIV/AIDS policy, Indigenous policies, and the representation of diverse women in STEM fields. Despite increased recognition that intersectionality-informed approaches are necessary to capture the complexity of people's lives, they have not yet permeated the field of public health.

References

Annandale, E., & Hunt, K. (Eds.). (2000). *Gender inequalities in health*. Buckingham: Open University Press.

Bowleg, L. (2012). The problem with the phrase women and minorities: Intersectionality—An important theoretical framework for public health. *American Journal of Public Health, 102*(7), 1267–1273.

Buettgen, A., Hardie, S., Wicklund, E., Jean-François, K. M., & Alimi, S. (2018). *Understanding the intersectional forms of discrimination impacting persons with disabilities*. Ottawa: Government of Canada's Social Development Partnerships Program – Disability Component. Canadian Centre on Disability Studies.

Bunjun, B. (2010). Feminist organizations and intersectionality: Contesting hegemonic feminism. *Atlantis, 34*(2), 115–126.

Centre of Excellence for Women's Health [CEWH]. (2020). Framework for gender transformative health promotion. In *Gender transformative health promotion course*. Retrieved from http://bccewh.bc.ca/webinars-and-courses/courses/gender-transformative-health-promotion-course/unit-1-what-is-gender-transformative-health-promotion/framework-for-gender-transformative-health-promotion/

Chan, C. D., Steen, S., Howard, L. C., & Ali, A. I. (2019). Disentangling the complexities of queer theory and intersectionality theory: Research paradigms and insights for social justice. In *Research methods for social justice and equity in education* (pp. 59–70). Cham: Palgrave Macmillan.

Collins, P. H. (1990). *Black feminist thought: Knowledge, consciousness, and the politics of empowerment*. New York: Routledge.

Collins, P. H., & Bilge, S. (2016). *Intersectionality*. John Wiley & Sons.

Crenshaw, K. (1989). Mapping the margins: Intersectionality, identity politics, and violence against women of color. *Stanford Law Review, 43*, 1241.

Darmstadt, G. L., Heise, L., Gupta, G. R., Henry, S., Cislaghi, B., Greene, M. E., et al. (2019). Why now for a series on gender equality, norms, and health? *The Lancet, 393*(10189), 2374–2377.

Dworkin, S. L., & Barker, G. (2019). Gender-transformative approaches to engaging men in reducing gender-based violence: A response to Brush & Miller's "Trouble in Paradigm". *Violence Against Women, 25*(14), 1657–1671.

Dworkin, S. L., Fleming, P. J., & Colvin, C. J. (2015). The promises and limitations of gender-transformative health programming with men: Critical reflections from the field. *Culture, Health & Sexuality, 17*(sup2), 128–143.

EuroHealthNet. (2017). *Making the link: Gender equality and health*. Policy Préci. Retrieved from https://eurohealthnet.eu/sites/eurohealthnet.eu/files/publications/PP_Gender_Digital%20Version.pdf

Fehrenbacher, A., & Patel, D. (2020). Translating the theory of intersectionality into quantitative and mixed methods for empirical gender transformative research on health. *Culture, Health & Sexuality, 22*(sup1), 145–160.

Fleming, P. J., Lee, J. G., & Dworkin, S. L. (2014). "Real men don't": Constructions of masculinity and inadvertent harm in public health interventions. *American Journal of Public Health, 104*(6), 1029–1035.

George, A. S., Amin, A., de Abreu Lopes, C. M., & Ravindran, T. S. (2020). Structural determinants of gender inequality: Why they matter for adolescent girls' sexual and reproductive health. *BMJ, 368*, L6985. https://doi.org/10.1136/bmj.l6985

Gkiouleka, A., Huijts, T., Beckfield, J., & Bambra, C. (2018). Understanding the micro and macro politics of health: Inequalities, intersectionality & institutions-A research agenda. *Social Science & Medicine, 200*, 92–98.

Greaves, L., Pederson, A., & Poole, N. (Eds.). (2014). *Making it better: Gender transformative health promotion*. Toronto: Canadian Scholars' Press.

Grzanka, P., & Grzanka, P. R. (2018). *Intersectionality: A foundations and frontiers reader*. Routledge.

Gupta, G. R. (2000). *Gender, sexuality, and HIV/AIDS: The what, the why, and the how*. Washington, D.C.: International Center for Research on Women (ICRW).

Hancock, A. M. (2016). *Intersectionality: An intellectual history*. Oxford University Press.

Hankivsky, O. (2014). *Intersectionality 101*. The Institute for Intersectionality Research & Policy, SFU.

Hankivsky, O., & Christoffersen, A. (2008). Intersectionality and the determinants of health: A Canadian perspective. *Critical Public Health, 18*(3), 271–283.

Hankivsky, O., Doyal, L., Einstein, G., Kelly, U., Shim, J., Weber, L., & Repta, R. (2017). The odd couple: Using biomedical and intersectional approaches to address health inequities. *Global Health Action, 10*(sup2), 1326686. https://doi.org/10.1080/16549716.2017.1326686

Hankivsky, O., Grace, D., Hunting, G., Ferlatte, O., Clark, N., Fridkin, A., & Laviolette, T. (2012). Intersectionality-based policy analysis. In *An intersectionality-based policy analysis framework* (pp. 33–45). Vancouver, BC: Institute for Intersectionality Research & Policy, SFU.

Hawkes, S., Allotey, P., Sy Elhadj, A., Clark, J., & Horton, R. (2020). The Lancet Commission on Gender and Global Health. Comment. *The Lancet, 396*, 521–522. Retrieved from https://www.thelancet.com/action/showPdf?pii=S0140-6736%2820%2931547-6

Hawkes, S., & Buse, K. (2013). Gender and global health: Evidence, policy, and inconvenient truths. *The Lancet, 381*(9879), 1783–1787.

Heard, E., Fitzgerald, L., Wigginton, B., & Mutch, A. (2020). Applying intersectionality theory in health promotion research and practice. *Health Promotion International, 35*(4), 866–876. https://doi.org/10.1093/heapro/daz080

Heise, L., Greene, M. E., Opper, N., Stavropoulou, M., Harper, C., Nascimento, M., et al. (2019). Gender inequality and restrictive gender norms: Framing the challenges to health. *The Lancet, 393*(10189), 2440–2454.

Hillenbrand, E., Karim, N., Mohanraj, P., & Wu, D. (2015). *Measuring gender-transformative change: A review of literature and promising practices*. Care USA Working Paper. Retrieved from https://care.org/wp-content/uploads/2020/05/working_paper_aas_gt_change_measurement_fa_lowres.pdf

Horgan, S. A., Chen, S. P., Tuininga, T., & Stuart, H. (2020). Taking a closer look at gender-transformative health promotion programming as a vehicle for addressing gender-based inequities in health and care. *Global Health Promotion, 27*(3), 92–102. https://doi.org/10.1177/1757975919864109

Kapilashrami, A., & Hankivsky, O. (2018). Intersectionality and why it matters to global health. *The Lancet, 391*(10140), 2589–2591.

Kapilashrami, A., Hill, S., & Meer, N. (2015). What can health inequalities researchers learn from an intersectionality perspective? Understanding social dynamics with an inter-categorical approach? *Social Theory & Health, 13*(3–4), 288–307.

Krieger, N. (2014). Discrimination and health inequities. *International Journal of Health Services, 44*(4), 643–710.

Martinez, E., & Wu, D. (2009). *CARE SII women's empowerment framework summary sheet*. Atlanta: CARE International.

Mendell, A., Dyck, L., Ndumbe-Eyoh, S., & Morisson, V. (2012). *Tools and approaches for assessing and supporting public health action on the social determinants of health and health equity*. NCCDH & NCCHPP. Retrieved from http://www.ncchpp.ca/docs/Equity_Tools_NCCDH-NCCHPP.pdf

Morgan, M. (2014). Measuring gender transformative change. In *CGIAR Research Program on Aquatic Agricultural Systems* (Program Brief: AAS-2014-41). Penang, Malaysia. Retrieved from https://www.worldfishcenter.org/content/measuring-gender-transformative-change

National Collaborating Centre for Healthy Public Policy [NCCHPP]. (2015). *Health inequalities and intersectionality*. Retrieved from http://www.ncchpp.ca/docs/2015_Ineg_Ineq_Intersectionnalite_En.pdf

Palència, L., Malmusi, D., & Borrell, C. (2014). SOPHIE: Evaluating the impact of structural policies on health inequalities and their social determinants and fostering change. In *Incorporating intersectionality in evaluation of policy impacts on health equity: A quick guide*. Retrieved from http://www.sophie-project.eu/pdf/Guide_intersectionality_SOPHIE.pdf

Pederson, A., Greaves, L., & Poole, N. (2014). Gender-transformative health promotion for women: A framework for action. *Health Promotion International, 30*(1), 140–150.

Peretz, T., Lehrer, J., & Dworkin, S. L. (2020). Impacts of Men's gender-transformative personal narratives: A qualitative evaluation of the Men's story project. *Men and Masculinities, 23*(1), 104–126.

Plan International. (2019). *Our gender transformative approach: Tackling the root causes of gender inequality*. Retrieved from https://plan-international.org/eu/blog-alex-munive-gender-transformative-approach

Rolleri, L. A. (2014). *Gender transformative programming in adolescent reproductive and sexual health: Definitions, strategies, and resources*. New York: ACT for Youth Center of Excellence, Bronfenbrenner Center for Translational Research. Retrieved from http://www.actforyouth.net/resources/pm/pm_gender4_0114.pdf

Rosenthal, L. (2016). Incorporating intersectionality into psychology: An opportunity to promote social justice and equity. *American Psychologist, 71*(6), 474.

Roth, J. (2018). Feminism otherwise: Intersectionality beyond Occidentalism. *InterDisciplines, 8*(2). https://doi.org/10.4119/indi-1047

Rottach, E., Schuler, S. R., & Hardee, K. (2009). *Gender perspectives improve reproductive health outcomes: New evidence*. Population Reference Bureau. Retrieved from http://www.igwg.org/igwg_media/genderperspectives.pdf

Ruane-McAteer, E., Amin, A., Hanratty, J., Lynn, F., van Willenswaard, K. C., Reid, E., et al. (2019). Interventions addressing men, masculinities and gender equality in sexual and reproductive health and rights: An evidence and gap map and systematic review of reviews. *BMJ Global Health, 4*(5), e001634.

Rutgers. (2018). *Rutger's Gender Transformative Approach Toolkit*. Retrieved from https://www.rutgers.international/sites/rutgersorg/files/PDF/GTA%20Factsheet.pdf

Rutgers. (2020). *Gender transformative approach*. Rutgers, For Sexual and Reproductive Health and Rights. Retrieved from https://www.rutgers.international/GTA

Sen, G., & Östlin, P. (2007). *Unequal, unfair, ineffective and inefficient gender inequity in health: Why it exists and how we can change it*. Final Report to the WHO Commission on Social Determinants of Health. Retrieved from https://www.who.int/social_determinants/resources/csdh_media/wgekn_final_report_07.pdf?ua=1

Standing Committee on the Status of Women [SCSW]. (2016). *Implementing gender-based analysis plus in the Government of Canada*. Report of the Standing Committee on the Status of Women. Retrieved from https://www.ourcommons.ca/Content/Committee/421/FEWO/Reports/RP8355396/feworp04/feworp04-e.pdf

Status of Women Canada. (2018). *Government of Canada's Approach: GBA+*. Retrieved from https://cfc-swc.gc.ca/gba-acs/approach-approche-en.html

Stinson, J., Wolfson, L., & Poole, N. (2020). Technology-based substance use interventions: Opportunities for gender-transformative health promotion. *International Journal of Environmental Research and Public Health, 17*(3), 992.

Thomas, J. C., Sage, M., Dillenberg, J., & Guillory, V. J. (2002). A code of ethics for public health. *American Journal of Public Health, 92*, 1057–1059.

Trickett, E. J., Beehler, S., Deutsch, C., Green, L. W., Hawe, P., McLeroy, K., et al. (2011). Advancing the science of community-level interventions. *American Journal of Public Health, 101*(8), 1410–1419.

UN Women. (2020). *Counted and visible: Global conference on the measurement of gender equality, leave no one behind and intersecting inequalities*. Concept Note. Retrieved from https://data.unwomen.org/sites/default/files/inline-files/Global%20Conference%20on%20 Intersectionality%20-%20Concept%20note.pdf

Valdes, F. (1997). Foreword: Poised at the cusp: LatCrit theory outsider jurisprudence and Latina/o self-empowerment. *Harvard Latinx Law Review, 2*, 1.

Van Herk, K. A., Smith, D., & Andrew, C. (2011). Identity matters: Aboriginal mothers' experiences of accessing health care. *Contemporary Nurse, 37*(1), 57–68.

World Health Organization [WHO]. (2011). *Gender mainstreaming for health managers: A practical approach – Participant's notes*. Geneva: WHO.

World Health Organization [WHO]. (2020). *TDR intersectional gender research strategy: Building the science of solutions for all*. Geneva: WHO. https://apps.who.int/iris/bitstream/handle/1 0665/332288/9789240005068-eng.pdf

Chapter 13
Translation, Implementation and Engagement

Krystle van Hoof and Cara Tannenbaum

Introduction

Historically, the barriers to incorporating sex- and gender-based content and processes into public health policy and practice spanned a variety of issues. First, sex and gender were largely ignored during early development of the theory and practice of knowledge translation (also called knowledge transfer, mobilization and exchange) and implementation science, which evolved to speed up the natural diffusion of information across what the World Health Organization (WHO) calls the "know-do gap" (Pablos-Mendez & Shademani, 2006). Second, efforts in public health to close the know-do gap tended to follow an efficient one-size-fits-all population approach, without consideration of personal identity characteristics (Andermann et al., 2016). Third, while we have seen significant progress in recent years, the integration of sex and gender within evidence generation processes has been lacking in health research (Johnson et al., 2009). From basic science to clinical and population health research, female animals have been omitted from basic science experiments and women have been left out of clinical trials (Beery & Zucker, 2011). While regulations have driven an increase in women's inclusion in clinical research, there has not been a parallel increase in the disaggregation and analysis of data by sex and/or gender, making it challenging for public health officials to apply a sex and gender lens to evidence-informed policy and programme decision-making (Welch et al., 2017; Avery & Clark, 2016; Petkovic et al., 2018). However, with the integration of sex and gender on the rise in research, there are opportunities to ensure that knowledge used to inform public health includes sex and gender

K. van Hoof (✉)
Healthy Brains, Healthy Lives, McGill University, Montreal, QC, Canada

C. Tannenbaum
Faculty of Medicine, Université de Montréal, Montreal, QC, Canada

© Springer Nature Switzerland AG 2021   161
J. Gahagan, M. K. Bryson (eds.), *Sex- and Gender-Based Analysis in Public Health*, https://doi.org/10.1007/978-3-030-71929-6_13

considerations, in addition to other intersecting identity factors. Achieving this goal will require thorough engagement of stakeholders across research, policy and practice to ensure effective translation and implementation of evidence-based, equitable public health policies and programmes.

In this chapter, we discuss the rationale and methods for routinely incorporating sex and gender in public health knowledge translation and implementation processes. Throughout, we will provide examples and suggested positive ways forward.

Knowledge Translation and Implementation

The Canadian Institutes of Health Research defines knowledge translation as a dynamic and iterative process that includes synthesis, dissemination, exchange and ethically sound application of knowledge to improve health, provide more effective health services and products and strengthen the healthcare system (Canadian Institutes of Health Research, 2012). Lavis et al. identify a five-part framework for achieving effective knowledge translation (2003). We encourage adaptation of Lavis et al.'s framework to sex and gender by posing the following five questions: (1) What sex and gender information should be transferred to decision-makers (the message)?; (2) To whom should research knowledge be transferred (are there sex- and/or gender-specific target audiences)?; (3) By whom should research knowledge be transferred (sex and/or gender of the messenger)?; (4) How should sex- and/or gender-related research knowledge be transferred (the knowledge-transfer processes and supporting communications infrastructure)?; (5) With what effect should research knowledge be transferred (evaluation of sex and/or gender outcomes)?

The Message

The first of these components, the message, must include sex- and/or gender-based evidence. Systematic reviews represent one of the key ways those working in public health obtain evidence (Grimshaw et al., 2012). Established in 2005, the Cochrane Sex/Gender Methods Group fosters the integration of sex- and gender-based analysis in research synthesis and more recently developed a planning tool to guide others wishing to integrate sex and gender into systematic reviews (Sex/Gender Methods Group, 2019; Doull et al., 2011). The tool recommends reviewing whether sex and/or gender are relevant to the question under study, whether sex and/or gender differences may be expected and whether the inclusion or exclusion criteria have sex- or gender-related biases, addressing the possibility of differences in outcomes by sex and/or gender, ensuring that the data extraction sheet collects results separately by sex and/or gender and analysing and reporting the results by sex and/or gender.

As systematic reviews rely on previously published trials, progress to consider and report sex- and gender-related considerations has been slow but promising. Of 1373 systematic reviews published by Cochrane and Campbell between August 2016 and July 2017, 27% included mention of sex and/or gender in their results, and 14% included sex and/or gender in the discussion section (Petkovic et al., 2018). Given that funding agencies and journal editors have become more stringent in their requirements for sex and gender reporting, we anticipate a steep growth in the number of systematic reviews that incorporate sex and gender evidence. The next step to consider then is how to use this evidence to craft a sex- and/or gender-effective message.

The easiest way to emphasize sex and gender in a message is by explicitly referring to specific population groups. Instead of entitling a report or policy brief "Human Papilloma Vaccination Rates", call it "Human Papilloma Vaccination Rates Among Adolescent Males and Females", or "in Adult Men and Women", or "in Men Who Have Sex With Men." Drawing attention to specific populations raises awareness of the need to understand and tailor programmes accordingly.

An example of a successful gender-sensitive public health knowledge-translation campaign is Sweden's "Gender-Balanced Snow-Clearing Policy" (Criado-Perez, 2019). Notice the reference to gender balance in the name of the policy. By asking whether pedestrian injuries in winter differed by sex, Swedish municipal authorities discovered that two-thirds of injuries occurred in women who slipped and fell on snowy or icy surfaces. The majority of injuries were sustained by older women, women with unpaid work, women accompanying small children to school and women with lower socioeconomic status who did not own cars but walked to take public transportation. Accordingly, the first streets to be snow-cleaned were the large arteries leading into the business areas, generally serving rich men with cars and high-paying occupations. Smaller streets, sidewalks and bike paths were cleared afterwards. Once analysts applied a gender lens to the problem, they realized the order in which the streets were cleaned needed to be reversed. When small streets and lanes were snow-cleared first, pedestrian accidents went down by half. The message itself was as clear as the sidewalks: snow-clearing must be gender-balanced because women are overrepresented among those susceptible to slipping and falling on icy surfaces due to gender-related activities.

The way the message is crafted is the first building block for evidence-informed decision-making in public health that accounts for sex and gender. The message should be founded on relevant sex and gender data and, if possible, be solution-oriented. Once the evidence is available and the message clearly presented, it still must be made accessible to those who can understand and use it to improve public health outcomes in equitable ways. For this reason, it is generally recommended to engage members of the target audience in crafting the message. A recent toolkit published by the World Health Organization, *Incorporating Intersectional Gender Analysis into Research on Infectious Diseases of Poverty* (World Health Organization, 2020), provides concrete advice for integrating gender and intersectional factors to stakeholder engagement in implementation and knowledge translation.

The Target Audience

The target audience is the intended recipient of the message. The choice of language used, the strength of persuasion of the communication strategy and the way promotional information is processed can have a differential effect based on the sex- and gender-related characteristics of the target audience. Furthermore, some target audiences may be more difficult to reach, due to stigma or other barriers.

Imagine we wanted to develop a suicide-reduction campaign for older men. Alternatively, what if our target audience were transgender individuals? Would the knowledge translation strategy shift for two-spirit Indigenous persons? One could envision tailored approaches with a different choice of language, reach and penetration, depending on the target population.

An initiative to promote healthy body weights in youth might target boys and girls through school-based programmes, or alternatively through media that targets gendered caregiving roles, such as parenthood magazines. If there were concern about eating disorders, one might want to target specific populations such as ballet dancers, gymnasts or fashion models. Gendered social networks often connect members of the target audience, particularly through social media among youth and gender-diverse communities. To prevent obesity, a suite of physical activity options could be developed to appeal across the full spectrum of youth gender identities.

What is important when planning tailored approaches is to be wary not to fall into the trap of inadvertently reinforcing stereotypes about the target audience. Anti-smoking campaigns during pregnancy targeted only at the pregnant mother unwittingly underscore that the mother alone is responsible for the baby's health. A more transformative approach would be to advertise that the parents, together, should watch out for the health of their infant and quit smoking together (Greaves, 2014).

The Messenger

Trusting the messenger is key for ensuring uptake of the message and may have gendered ramifications. Asking sex and gender questions about beliefs surrounding the messenger can elucidate enablers and barriers to the adoption of complex behavioural interventions. For instance, a qualitative study examined vaccine hesitancy among Somali women in Minnesota (Pratt et al., 2019). Some women expressed mistrust of government, claiming that government officials were cold and unfeeling during forced vaccination upon arrival to the United States. The women perceived getting shots was necessary because they were dirty and carrying diseases. Furthermore, there was a power differential, with government having the right to deny them citizenship. Other women valued the freedom to choose. They recalled not having a choice before they immigrated to the United States. When their parents told them to do what the doctor said, they previously did not have a say in the matter.

It follows, therefore, that warnings by government, or even requests by doctors for Somali women to vaccinate their children, might impede uptake due to historical mistrust and negative lived experiences. Careful thought should go into selection of a key opinion leader to deliver the public health message, preferably one who shares identity characteristics with the target audience.

The Process

The process of knowledge translation benefits from the application of implementation science (also called dissemination or implementation research). Implementation science has been defined as an area of research that aims to determine "what works, for whom, under what contextual conditions and is it scalable in equitable ways" (Edwards & Barker, 2014). A relatively young and emergent field, implementation science's original concern was primarily with the implementation of evidence-based health-care practice (Foy et al., 2015). However, in more recent years, the field has expanded to include public health—as evidenced by the 2015 change in scope of the field's primary journal, *Implementation Science*, which added evidence-based population health to the journal's mandate (Foy et al., 2015). The integration of sex and gender in the field of implementation science is still in its infancy, but guidelines have been published and uptake is becoming more mainstream (Tannenbaum et al., 2016).

The academic discourse and practice of incorporating sex and gender in implementation science stands to learn from the effective implementation of these approaches in health promotion work out of the Global South. The World Health Organization (WHO) produced a review of interventions that engaged men and boys and found that gender-transformative interventions, which included deliberate discussion of gender and masculinity and clear efforts to transform harmful gender norms, were more effective than those that did not (World Health Organization, 2011; Barker et al., 2007). In contrast to a gender-blind approach, which aims to treat everyone the same but may actually have unintended consequences that worsen gender equity, a gender-transformative approach aims to address the underlying causes of gender inequity in addition to a particular health outcome (Tannenbaum et al., 2016).

One area that has paid particular attention not only to incorporating gender but also gender-transformative approaches is that of HIV/AIDS prevention initiatives (Ghosn et al., 2018; Amin, 2015). The rate of gender-transformative interventions in the area of HIV/AIDS has been found to be higher (60%) than the rate among gender-based violence (GBV) interventions (46%), and the effectiveness of interventions in the area of HIV/AIDS was also rated higher than in GBV (42% effective vs. 25% effective) (World Health Organization, 2011). These data give some indication that the area of HIV/AIDS programme implementation is integrating gender and gender-transformative approaches effectively and is somewhat ahead of other areas in this regard (World Health Organization, 2011). Indeed, the very notion of assessing health interventions on the basis of how they engage critically with gender came out of global efforts to address HIV/AIDS. The origins of the WHO Gender-Responsive Assessment Scale, including the concept of gender-transformative approaches, was a speech given by Geeta Rao Gupta in a plenary presentation on 12 July, 2000, at the XIII International AIDS Conference in Durban, South Africa (Gupta, 2000).

When using participatory and collaborative or integrated knowledge translation research approaches, it is important to consider the sex and gender of the researchers and knowledge users (Banister & Begoray, 2019). Do gender relations play a role in the dynamic that ensues, and if so, how? Similarly, how might gender relations as a function of dyads or interpersonal dynamics within an organization, community, workplace or institution influence the outcome of the intervention?

Finally, a key tenet of implementation science is adaptation to local context. The gendered nature of context usually emerges as a function of the target audience and setting. Recognition of gendered contexts and how the message might need to be adapted to this context are critical to achieving scale-up and spread of successful public interventions. Making sure that the practice or policy under consideration aligns with the priorities of the target group or setting increases the likelihood of meaningful adoption and change.

Evaluation

An approach for evaluating both changes in outcome and changes to harmful gender norms is required to effectively integrate gender-transformative approaches into the implementation of public health interventions. The WHO evaluation of interventions that engage men and boys, referenced earlier, looked at changes in knowledge, attitudes and behaviours (self-reported as well as corroborated by others) to determine if gender transformation was taking place (World Health Organization, 2011). A 2015 report from UKAiD included indicators that looked at changes to attitude, intentions, practices and outcomes and perceptions of gender norms to evaluate progress on gender-transformative change (Overseas Development Institute, 2015). In addition to evaluating change at the individual level, indicators to measure change in overarching patriarchal structures in a community or culture should be considered, as these reproduce and propagate gender norms at the individual level (Ruane-McAteer et al., 2018).

Evaluation also involves asking how gender roles, gender identity, gender relations and institutionalized gender influence the way in which an implementation strategy works, for whom, under what circumstances and why, or how programmes work within and across sexes, genders and other diversity characteristics and in what circumstances. Finally, findings from the evaluation should be disaggregated and reported by sex or gender groups. In order to inform future initiatives, it is critical to report whether there are similar effects or differences.

Conclusion

Knowledge translation and implementation will be more effective if sex and gender are considered across the five key components of the message, the target audience, the messenger, the process and the evaluation strategy. Engaging members of the target audience early in the knowledge translation planning process will ensure better adaptation to gendered contexts and enhanced buy-in from those who stand to benefit most. Public health may apply to populations, but only by taking sex, gender and other identity characteristics into consideration will true social impact be achieved at the individual level.

References

Amin, A. (2015). Addressing gender inequalities to improve the sexual and reproductive health and wellbeing of women living with HIV. *Journal of International AIDS Society, 18*(Suppl 5), 20302.

Andermann, A., et al. (2016). Evidence for Health II: Overcoming barriers to using evidence in policy and practice. *Health Research Policy and Systems, 14*, 17.

Avery, E., & Clark, J. (2016). Sex-related reporting in randomised controlled trials in medical journals. *Lancet, 388*(10062), 2839–2840.

Banister, E. M., & Begoray, D. L. (2019). Reflections on gender relations in an Indigenous female adolescent sexual health literacy program. In *What a difference sex and gender make: A gender, sex and health research casebook*. Available online at http://www.cihr-irsc.gc.ca/e/44734. html#aii. Accessed 10 June 2019.

Barker, G., et al. (2007). *Engaging men and boys in changing gender-based inequity in health: Evidence from programme interventions*. WHO.

Beery, A. K., & Zucker, I. (2011). Sex bias in neuroscience and biomedical research. *Neuroscience and Biobehavioral Reviews, 35*(3), 565–572.

Canadian Institutes of Health Research. (2012). *Guide to knowledge translation planning at CIHR: Integrated and end-of-grant approaches*. Canadian Institutes of Health Research.

Criado-Perez, C. (2019). *Invisible women: Data bias in a world designed for men* (pp. 31–32). New York: Abrams Press.

Doull, M., Runnels, V., Tudiver, S., & Boscoe, M. (2011). *Sex and gender in systematic reviews: Planning tool* (C.S.G.M. Group, Ed.). Available online at https://methods.cochrane.org/sites/ methods.cochrane.org.equity/files/public/uploads/SRTool_PlanningVersionSHORTFINAL. pdf. Accessed 8 June 2019.

Edwards, N., & Barker, P. M. (2014). The importance of context in implementation research. *JAIDS Journal of Acquired Immune Deficiency Syndromes, 67*, S157–S162.

Foy, R., et al. (2015). Implementation science: A reappraisal of our journal mission and scope. *Implementation Science, 10*, 51.

Ghosn, J., et al. (2018). Hiv. *Lancet, 392*(10148), 685–697.

Greaves, L. (2014). Can tobacco control be transformative? Reducing gender inequity and tobacco use among vulnerable populations. *International Journal of Environmental Research and Public Health, 11(1)*, 792–803.

Grimshaw, J. M., et al. (2012). Knowledge translation of research findings. *Implementation Science, 7*, 50.

Gupta, G. R. (2000). Gender, sexuality, and HIV/AIDS: The what, the why, and the how. *Canadian HIV/AIDS Policy & Law Review, 5*(4), 86–93.

Johnson, J. L., Greaves, L., & Repta, R. (2009). Better science with sex and gender: Facilitating the use of a sex and gender-based analysis in health research. *International Journal for Equity in Health, 8*, 14.

Lavis, J. N., Robertson, D., Woodside, J. M., McLeod, C. B., & Abelson, J. (2003). How can research organizations more effectively transfer research knowledge to decision makers? *Milbank Quarterly, 81*(2), 221–222.

Overseas Development Institute. (2015). *Changing gender norms: Monitoring and evaluating programmes and projects. Knowledge to action resource series 2015* (R. Marcus & C. Harper, Eds.). London.

Pablos-Mendez, A., & Shademani, R. (2006). Knowledge translation in global health. *The Journal of Continuing Education in the Health Professions, 26*(1), 81–86.

Petkovic, J., et al. (2018). Sex/gender reporting and analysis in Campbell and Cochrane systematic reviews: A cross-sectional methods study. *Systematic Reviews, 7*(1), 113.

Pratt, R., et al. (2019). "We are Muslims and these diseases don't happen to us": A qualitative study of the views of young Somali men and women concerning HPV immunization. *Vaccine, 37*, 2043–2050.

Ruane-McAteer, E., Hanratty, J., Lynn, F., Reid, E., Khosla, R., Amin, A., & Lohan, M. (2018). Protocol for a systematic review: Interventions addressing men, masculinities and gender equality in sexual and reproductive health: An evidence and gap map and systematic review of reviews. *Campbell Systematic Reviews, 14*, 1–24.

Sex/Gender Methods Group. (2019). *Why sex and gender matter in health research synthesis.* Cochrane Methods Equity. Available from https://methods.cochrane.org/equity/sex-and-gender-analysis

Tannenbaum, C., Greaves, L., & Graham, I. D. (2016). Why sex and gender matter in implementation research. *BMC Medical Research Methodology, 16*(1), 145.

Welch, V., et al. (2017). Reporting of sex and gender in randomized controlled trials in Canada: A cross-sectional methods study. *Research Integrity and Peer Review, 2*(1), 15.

World Health Organization. (2011). *Gender mainstreaming for health managers: A practical approach* (pp. 41–42). Geneva: WHO.

World Health Organization. (2020). *Incorporating intersectional gender analysis into research on infectious diseases of poverty: A toolkit for health researchers* (pp. 109–130). Geneva: WHO.

Index

© Springer Nature Switzerland AG 2021
J. Gahagan, M. K. Bryson (eds.), *Sex- and Gender-Based Analysis in Public Health*, https://doi.org/10.1007/978-3-030-71929-6

Printed in the United States
by Baker & Taylor Publisher Services